LESS
WE CAN

The Case for Less Government, More Liberty,
More Prosperity, and More Security

MARK GRANNIS

ISBN: 061562300X
ISBN-13: 9780615623009

Library of Congress Control Number: 2012936845
Thoroughfare Books
Chevy Chase, Maryland

Contents

Introduction

In 2010, the Libertarian Party of Maryland honored me with its nomination for the U.S. House of Representatives, representing Maryland's 8th District. During one midsummer campaign debate, the moderator asked me to begin with a short summary of libertarianism before moving on to the hot topics of the day. Ad libbing, I asked my listeners to raise their hands if I was the first libertarian they had ever seen in the flesh. *About half did so.* From that point on, I understood that my job wasn't really to make people vote for *me*; it was to make people vote for liberty.

As the 2012 campaign begins, I am once again the Libertarian Party's nominee, and it feels like I am already far ahead of where I began two years ago. Libertarianism has become familiar to many more voters. Ron Paul's very libertarian campaign for the Republican presidential nomination has been a golden opportunity to spread libertarian ideas to a much wider audience. Libertarian voices are also somewhat better represented in the media, thanks to television personalities like Judge Andrew Napolitano and John Stossel, as well as best-selling authors like Matt Welch and Nick Gillespie. The Libertarian Party is growing bigger and stronger nearly everywhere, and candidates in all parties seem much more eager to embrace libertarian language, if not always libertarian principles.

And yet the view from 2012 is far from rosy. Our political culture remains dominated by men and women who are addicted to coercion. The last two years have brought more war (undeclared by Congress, of course), more regulation, more public debt, and further erosion of our civil liberties. Instead of contenting themselves with attention to genuinely public problems (like, say, the Congress's inability to pay its bills, or the President's unwillingness to abide by the Constitution), the vast majority of our elected officials compete with one another to propose more and more coercive interference with private behavior. Who has time to pass a budget when there's such a pressing need to ban incandescent light bulbs? There is much work still to be done in making the case for liberty.

My six months as a first-time candidate in 2010 taught me many things, but the most important thing I learned is this: Campaigns are just as important as elections. Public discussion of political issues has independent value, no matter who wins. This is not to deny that it matters who wins; it matters a great deal. But if (as I believe) the winner of any given election usually reflects the voters' own attitudes back at them, then in the long run the health of the republic requires politicians who care more about articulating their principles than about winning an election. It is almost always from some once-small minority that majorities learn how to govern better.

Historically, this has been the mission of minor-party candidates like Libertarians. Certainly we hope to see Libertarians elected to office in far greater numbers than they are today. But that day will not come all at once, no matter how slick our campaign ads, how generous our donors, or how telegenic our candidates. We first need to change minds, to reawaken among ordinary citizens a real appreciation not just for the burdens of government, but for "the blessings of liberty." If we succeed in that task, the elections will take care of themselves. In that sense, winning is the goal of our efforts, but not the point.

It is in that spirit that I offer these essays from the campaign trail. Taken together, they offer not just a collection of issue positions but the elaboration of a consistent political philosophy, built on very old and very good ideas about the role government should play in our lives. Adapting the fundamental principles to national politics today, I attempt to give robust expression to the four main themes of my campaign: less government, more liberty, more prosperity, and more security. I hope the reader will find the essays helpful in thinking about the many policy questions we now must face.

PART I:

An Overview of the Main Issues

What the Wrong Track Looks Like

Anyone old enough to vote this year is old enough to remember

- a Democratic president with a Democratic Congress;
- a Republican president with a Democratic Congress;
- a Republican president with a Republican Congress; and
- a Democratic president with a Republican Congress.

Taken together, these four periods exhaust all the ways power can be split between the two major parties in Washington. What did all these periods have in common? Government got bigger.

That's a problem, not because government is always bad, but because the *proper* functions of government do not require it to be very big. Government today is big not primarily because of waste or indolence, but because we have asked it to do too many things. And now, thanks to both Democrats and Republicans, the relentless growth of our government has brought us to financial calamity.

Our government can't pay its bills, but it won't stop borrowing or spending. As a result, the government is currently headed for insolvency. Our economy badly needs jobs and investment from the private sector, but instead of encouraging private enterprise our elected officials continue to concentrate power and money in Washington. We need to change course, and we need to do it now.

The new course we should chart is not really new to people who know our history. It's actually a return to the values that made our country great. It's a return to individual liberty, limited government, economic freedom, and the good sense to mind our own business in military matters. That's the Libertarian way forward, and it's a way that the two major parties both abandoned years ago.

With government, less really is more.

Libertarian ideas offer the promise of a new start on a wide range of persistent social problems, from high unemployment in our cities to low test scores in our schools. But first, we have to address the debt crisis big government has created. We have to turn the ship around.

It won't be easy. In the near term, we need to fire Congress and put new people at the helm, people who actually believe in limited government and individual liberty. The incumbent Democrats and Republicans obviously don't.

More fundamentally, we need to forge a strong and durable political consensus against the knee-jerk impulse to offer a government "solution" as soon as any social problem is identified. We need to let our scaremongering officials know that we're perfectly capable of taking care of ourselves *and each other* without a federal bureaucracy for every facet of social life. If we re-elect people who have given us bad government, we're going to get more bad government. That's an outcome we literally can't afford.

The top policy priority for the next Congress should be to put our fiscal house in order, by eliminating federal programs that are unnecessary or unaffordable, and in many cases ineffective or even unconstitutional. That includes federal subsidies for agriculture, banking, carmakers, drug companies, energy companies, and so on through the alphabet. It includes the mountain of special favors that Democrats and Republicans alike have stuffed into the tax code for decades. It includes the bloated bureaucracies that have already made education and health care much more expensive than they would be in a free market. It includes much of our national security establishment, especially the parts that are operating outside the Constitution. I and other Libertarians have published budget proposals that show exactly how we can achieve these goals in just one year.

We also need to liberate our economy from the federal micromanagement that has imposed heavier and heavier burdens on existing businesses while discouraging the formation of new businesses. And we really can't get ourselves back to financial health unless we abandon the imperial designs that have led us to tragic miscalculations of our power and our interest in the Middle East. We need to embrace a non-interventionist foreign policy and shore up our civil liberties at home.

Finally, we need some common-sense political reforms to dismantle the various incumbency-protection mechanisms the two major parties have created at the federal level. That means term limits, redistricting reform, and fundamental tax reform—for starters. We should also adopt the "Downsize D.C." package of measures designed to clean up the legislative process. And under no circumstances should we let Congress enact any additional restrictions on political speech, because it's a safe bet that anything Congress passes will favor incumbents and make Congress less representative.

Balancing Our Budget

We have to shrink government,
whether we want to or not.

Since 2001, Democrats and Republicans alike, in Congress and in the White House, have borrowed and spent us into the worst economic conditions in living memory. The federal government borrows more than 40 cents out of every dollar it spends, piling up more debt at a truly alarming rate. A compliant Federal Reserve Bank prints enough money to keep interest rates as low as they can go, but still the government expects to pay $248 billion in interest on our national debt in Fiscal Year 2013. And even with this unprecedented amount of paper money sloshing through the financial system, unemployment remains stubbornly high and business investment remains depressingly low.

Then there's the matter of whom we're borrowing the money from. To some extent, we borrow it from foreign creditors, many of whom might become unreliable very suddenly as conditions worsen. But the real outrage is the amount we've borrowed from the future—from the very people who are finding it so difficult to find work as they try to enter the workforce today. It's no wonder these young people are deserting traditional Republicans and Democrats in droves.

Every candidate claims to be in favor of lower deficits, but most never make any serious attempt to achieve that result. The sad truth, though, is that even smaller deficits are not enough. *Any* deficit means we're piling up more debt, allowing our financial problems to get worse. That's why, in 2010, I teamed up with Ohio Libertarian Travis Irvine to produce a balanced budget for Fiscal Year 2012. Our budget would have eliminated the deficit already, and would have created rising surpluses in the years to come.

Here's how the Libertarian Balanced Federal Budget proposed to get the job done:

- *Over $900 billion in spending cuts.* Career politicians like to make ridiculously vague pledges to cut "waste, fraud, and abuse," but they rarely get specific; and when they do, the cuts never amount to very much. There was no such shilly-shallying in the Libertarian Balanced Federal Budget proposal. We went through the entire federal budget, agency by agency and program by program, to identify the agencies that could be consolidated, the programs that could be privatized or devolved to the states, and the functions that are simply not authorized by any reasonably faithful reading of the U.S. Constitution. We proposed to eliminate many programs we would want to end even if they were free, such as agricultural price supports and the federal "war on drugs." But we also proposed to eliminate some programs that might be wonderful to have if they were free, or even if we could afford their costs. We took no particular joy in proposing those cuts, but the fact is that no program is free and we simply cannot afford as much government as Congress has been authorizing.

- *No changes to Social Security or Medicare, with only minor changes to Medicaid.* Medicaid, which is largely funded by federal "block grants" to the states, was capped at 2010 levels under our budget, leaving the states fully in charge of deciding how much additional money to spend on that program—and also in charge of where to find the money. But we left Social Security and Medicare untouched, not because we thought those programs should continue to operate as they do today, but rather because we wanted to show that the budget *can* be balanced without injecting difficult issues like comprehensive entitlement reform into the process. (The same is true of comprehensive tax reform.) Republicans and Democrats seem to want us to believe that nothing constructive can be done about the budget unless we either increase tax rates significantly or completely restructure federal entitlement programs. That's just not true.

- *Over $414 billion from the elimination of corporate welfare and other gimmicky tax credits.* These tax credits proliferate under Democrats and Republicans alike because they're easy to hide in our sprawling 5.5-mllion-word tax code, and people don't usually pay a price at re-election time for giving away tax breaks. But the fact is that Congress routinely uses the tax code not just for the legitimate purpose of raising revenue, but for the less admirable purpose of throwing bones to politically connected interest groups. These "tax expenditures" amount to about $1 trillion per year. We cut out many of the worst offenders, adding $414 billion in revenues for 2012 even though we left current tax rates in place. Because some of the tax credits had to be phased out over periods as long as ten years, these simplifications of the tax code would have continued to grow federal revenue after 2012, totaling more than $7 trillion over the next ten years.

There is much more to say about this budget, and readers who want to learn more about it should consult Appendix A (our October 2010 press release describing the budget in more detail) and Appendix B (an agency-level summary of the entire budget). But note that if Libertarians had been elected to Congress in sufficient numbers last election, our budget would already have eliminated the federal budget deficit, and would have our national debt heading downward once again. Instead, the voters sent Republicans back to the House majority. The results (or lack thereof) speak for themselves.

Most Democrats and Republicans are simply not yet serious about fixing our fiscal situation. Due to the peculiarities of domestic politics, Democrats have an incentive to portray Republican budget proposals as dangerously austere, and Republicans generally don't fight that characterization because they want "credit" with their base for having made a bold proposal. For parallel reasons, Republicans portray Democratic budget proposals as profligately generous toward the poor, and Democrats don't fight that characterization either.

This year, Republican presidential candidate Ron Paul has proposed a budget very much like the one Travis Irvine and I proposed in 2010, and Libertarian presidential candidate Gary Johnson has proposed an even more ambitious plan. Having two serious presidential candidates release detailed budget proposals represents a big step in the right direction. But if we really want to see either budget enacted, we need to send Libertarians to Congress.

Restoring Our Civil Liberties

*Libertarians support civil liberties,
no matter who is in power.*

Since 2001, Presidents Bush and Obama have claimed the power to spy on U.S. citizens without warrants, detain U.S. citizens without charges, and imprison and even execute U.S. citizens without trials. Whatever one may think of the citizens involved in any individual case, as a lawyer I know too well how dangerous these precedents are for our liberties. We need representatives in Congress who appreciate the important role of civil liberties in maintaining our constitutional order, and who will call out a president of either party who violates his oath by making such aggressively unconstitutional claims.

The defense of our civil liberties should start with a staunch refusal to let government regulate our political speech in any way—including the regulation of campaign finances. No one in government should be in the position of deciding how much political speech is the right amount, or which kinds should be allowed. The first amendment says "Congress shall make no law . . . abridging the freedom of speech . . . ." There might be close cases in interpreting those words, but a law by which current officeholders try to regulate the speech of prospective challengers isn't one of them.

We should support the second amendment as strongly as we support the first. States should have the primary role in firearm regulation, and federal legislation should be limited to making sure that citizens who responsibly and legally exercise their second-amendment rights do not forfeit those federal rights when they cross state lines.

We must reverse the steady expansion of government eavesdropping. It has been over 25 years since Congress made any serious attempt to protect the privacy of electronic communications. That legislation was drafted in a world with brick-sized mobile phones (and not very many of them) and virtually no e-mail. It's not quite true to say the Internet didn't exist back then, but practically no one used it and people certainly didn't store personal information "in the cloud." Since that time, Congress has repeatedly acted to make sure telecom networks incorporate the eavesdropping *capabilities* that law enforcement agencies want, but Congress has made no comparable effort to update the *limits* on government eavesdropping. If most Americans today knew how vulnerable they now are to warrantless electronic snooping by the government, they would be horrified. This has got to change.

We have to start sticking up for the rights of the accused. Too many politicians act as if the police never make any mistakes and all criminal defendants are "guilty of something," even if it's not the crime with which they are charged. Part of the problem is that Congress has passed so many Draconian criminal statutes—to which the bureaucracy has added even more Draconian regulations—that nearly all of us *are* "guilty of something"—which gives the government the power to come after us almost at random, potentially shutting down innocent businesses based on mere suspicion. At the same time, we keep watering down the procedural protections that we've relied on literally *for centuries* to keep powerful government officials from using criminal prosecutions as weapons against political enemies. In 2011, we gave the military the authority to imprison U.S. citizens without a trial—in fact, without any criminal charges or any right to counsel. King George III didn't even have that power, and we called him a tyrant.

We need to get government out of the business of defining who can be married to whom. Most of the people on both sides of the "same-sex marriage" issue share the (usually unexamined) belief that government should decide. I say we should privatize marriage. Marriage is a voluntary, intimate, and often religious association between people. As such, it is none of the state's business. Certainly it is none of Congress's business.

Finally, I believe we need to return the difficult issue of abortion to the states so that each state can make its own determination of how to accommodate the rights of mothers and the rights of unborn children. This is an issue on which many Libertarians differ, because the very first question we need to resolve is whether there is one life at stake or two. But because I believe there are two lives involved, I believe each life deserves to be protected from any physical harm caused by the other. I recognize that many good people disagree, and in some states they may be in the majority. But the federal Constitution simply does not settle this issue, and we should restore the states' autonomy over abortion regulation.

Liberating Our Economy

*Prosperity is what free people choose
and what free people create.*

Real prosperity can't be counterfeited. You can't get prosperity by printing money. You can't get prosperity by creating a Federal Prosperity Agency or appointing a Prosperity Czar. And you sure can't get prosperity by taxing away the profits of small businesses to subsidize the losses of big businesses.

Prosperity is a byproduct of liberty. Free people produce abundance: abundance of food, clothing, energy, medicine, and other things that satisfy human want. Free people invented the steam engine, the light bulb, the telephone, the airplane, and the antibiotic. And if we want innovation and abundance to continue, we know that our liberty has got to continue.

There's a paradox here: When the government leaves us alone, real prosperity emerges from the individual choices of hard-working Americans who just want to be left alone. But when the government tries to take on the job of producing prosperity, we get what we have today: ruinous taxation, reckless spending, staggering unemployment, and a sagging dollar.

The most important element in a Libertarian program for liberating our economy is to *stay out of the way*. There are, however, some particular excesses from decades of government meddling that richly deserve legislative attention so that they can be repealed:

- *Stop overspending*. The government is currently violating the Hippocratic Oath ("First, do no harm"), the Rule of Holes ("When you're in a hole, stop digging"), and countless other cultural treasures of common sense by acting extremely aggressively to make our economy worse. The aggressive fiscal and monetary policies distort savings, investment, and consumption, and will most likely either fall flat or create new bubbles that will inevitably have to burst sometime in the future. Our mounting debts threaten the stability of our financial system as well as our political system. This all needs to stop.

- *Reform the tax system*. I discuss this more fully elsewhere, but it is hard to overemphasize how important fundamental tax reform is. To pick just one example, one of the main reasons our health care system was so lousy before Obamacare made it worse is because of tax deductions the government blessed back in the 1950s. The government uses tax goodies to nudge people into doing what the government thinks best. But micromanagement of individual decisions through the tax code is essentially a soft form of central planning. Like all attempts at central planning, it is doomed to distort private incentives and misallocate economic resources. Our incredibly detailed tax code embodies all the very worst tendencies of government to interfere with free-market outcomes in ways that make us all worse off.

- *Deregulate and decriminalize business.* Once a representative has been in Congress long enough to become a know-it-all, it is very hard for him to avoid reaching for the bluntest tool in the shop: federal criminal statutes. Between 1998 and 2007, the number of federal crimes on the books increased by 50%, and many of these statutes are used to prosecute people who are simply conducting legitimate business transactions without a shred of criminal intent. According to a 2010 story in the Washington Examiner, the 109th Congress (2005-2006) proposed 446 new crimes "that did not involve violence, firearms, drugs and drug trafficking, pornography, or immigration violations." My guess is that most normal people would have a hard time coming up with 10 real crimes that don't involve violence, guns, drugs, sex, or immigration, let alone 10 new crimes that didn't already exist before 2005. What are we to make of 446 new proposals for criminal prohibition—more than four a week? What's the matter with the people in Congress?

Defending Our Freedom

Our interventions in foreign conflicts
make us less secure and less prosperous.

Libertarian thinkers tend to regard defense of person and property as the main reason governments exist. Consequently, Libertarians support a standing military strong enough to defend the United States against aggression. Libertarians object, however, to policies that cast the United States in the role of global policeman.

It is not that Libertarians are indifferent to the spread of representative self-government. The Libertarian Party platform includes ringing affirmations of the rights of people everywhere to self-determination, representative government, and equality before the law. The platform also includes a powerful condemnation of terrorism, including terrorism committed by governments as well as by political or revolutionary groups. Libertarians also support free trade with all nations.

Yet Libertarians take the "non-interventionist" view that we have no right to use force against the people of any country that is not attacking us. According to this philosophy, trade, diplomacy, and a strong defense are all good; attempts to influence other nations by our friendship and by our example are also good; but military campaigns on foreign soil to make nations that have not attacked us see things our way are bad because they invade the liberty of others in a way that we ourselves would find intolerable. Besides these moral claims, Libertarians also believe that a foreign policy of worldwide readiness to intervene (and to defend the countries in which we garrison our troops) is as economically unsustainable as all previous attempts at global empire.

Some people (mainly Republicans) persist in describing Libertarians as "isolationists" because they tend to oppose foreign invasions. These charges betray an implicit but unmistakable bias toward war that is anything but conservative. And no less an authority than Sen. Robert A. Taft—known then as "Mr. Republican"—wrote in 1951

> that the overriding purpose of all American foreign policy should be the maintenance of the liberty and the peace of the people of the United States, so that they may achieve that intellectual and material improvement which is their genius and in which they can set an example for all people. By that example we can do an even greater service to mankind than we can by billions of material assistance—and more than we can ever do by war.

Taft acknowledged a "natural desire to bring freedom to others throughout the world," but pointed out that "the forcing of any special brand of freedom and democracy on a people, whether they want it or not, by the brute force of war will be a denial of those very democratic principles which we are striving to advance." He also recognized that the enormous economic costs of warfare posed a serious risk that the country might be weakened not by an external threat but by a self-inflicted economic wound:

> Just as our nation can be destroyed by war it can also be destroyed by a political or economic policy at home which destroys liberty or breaks down the fiscal and economic structure of the United States. We cannot adopt a foreign policy which gives away all of our people's earnings or imposes such a tremendous burden on the individual American as, in effect, to destroy his incentive and his ability to increase production and productivity in his standard of living. We cannot assume a financial burden in our foreign policy so great that it threatens liberty at home.

In 2008 it was easy to believe that Republicans needed to hear Taft's message more than Democrats did. But the unexpectedly bellicose presidency of Barack Obama—and the glee with which congressional Democrats have ceded to him their constitutional authority over matters of war and peace—make clear that this is yet another bipartisan failing. Members of the Party of Jefferson may wish to reflect on what Jefferson's closest ally, James Madison, said about war:

> Of all the enemies to public liberty war is, perhaps, the most to be dreaded, because it comprises and develops the germ of every other. War is the parent of armies; from these proceed debts and taxes; and armies, and debts, and taxes are the known instruments for bringing the many under the domination of the few . . . . No nation could preserve its freedom in the midst of continual warfare.

"Continual warfare." Isn't that exactly what we have had since 2001? Today's politicians tell us that continual warfare is necessary for our survival. James Madison thought it was *incompatible with our survival.* I'm with Madison.

The founders knew the difference between a republic and an empire. They didn't write any nonsense about making the world safe for democracy or ridding the world of evil-doers or even about protecting our vital interests overseas. They knew where our vital interests were.

It is high time for Congress to reclaim its constitutional authority over the decision to make war on other nations, and rein in the imperial overreach that is contributing so substantially to our problems. For starters, the open-ended resolutions authorizing the use of force in Afghanistan and Iraq should be amended to phase out the extraordinary "9/14 powers"—the phrase is Eli Lake's—that Congress gave President Bush three days after the 9/11 attacks. As Lake pointed out in Reason Magazine, "Just as President Bush said the 9/14 resolutions gave him the wartime powers to detain, interrogate, capture, and kill terrorists all over the world, so too does President Obama." It is the authority on which the Obama Justice Department has based its policies on military detention, and more recently, assassination. Such open-ended authorizations should be terminated or sunsetted before they become, by default, a permanent alteration of our system of constitutional checks and balances.

Welcoming Legal Immigration

Reducing illegal immigration requires
less government, not more.

We have two serious immigration problems in this country: not enough legal immigration, and too much illegal immigration. We can eliminate the first problem easily, mostly by getting government out of the way. But we need to be realistic about how much government can do to stop illegal immigration.

We'll never get legal immigration right unless we start from the premise that the immigration of peaceful and productive people into this country is good for us. We must never make the mistake of thinking that immigrants who come here seeking better lives are somehow taking something away from those of us who were born here. Our economy is not like a pie that can only be cut into so many slices. Our economy is dynamic; the pie grows whenever we add productive talent to our economy. Everyone who wants to make the pie bigger by working hard for himself and his family should be welcome here. That's true not only of the Alexander Graham Bells, and Albert Einsteins, and Sergey Brins who have contributed so much to our society, but also of the millions who labor in obscurity in fields and factories across the country. Immigration of peaceful and productive people is good for us.

That means we should clear away obstacles to legal immigration by peaceful, productive people and instead welcome them and their contributions into our society. The good news here is that government can do this. We can and should:

- *Create more visa opportunities for the kinds of immigrants we particularly want to attract.* Skilled workers, gifted students, and entrepreneurs are all obvious places to start, but the truth is that there is *no* reason why any peaceful person who is willing to enter on the express condition that he or she will not be eligible for public assistance should not be admitted.

- *Eliminate per-country ceilings on legal immigration.* Under current law, no more than 7 percent of some visas for skilled workers can be issued to applicants from any one country. That means it is much, much harder for skilled workers to get here from India or China than from, say, Cameroon. As we've seen, the unintended consequence of barring Chinese workers from coming over here to find jobs is that the jobs often end up getting sent to China where the workers are.

- *Reform our tax code to bring immigrants into the tax base.* Replacing our progressive income tax with a sales tax would eliminate any concern about immigrants enjoying the benefits of our society without paying taxes. Even illegal immigrants pay sales taxes.

Some people worry that, even though immigration is *generally* good for us, it is possible to have too much of it. These people tend to worry not just about economic effects but about cultural effects as well: the existence of large and unassimilated ethnic communities who may be less accustomed, or even less committed, to the institutions of self-government. But note that even people who worry about "too much" immigration in total should prefer to give those who might otherwise enter illegally an incentive to come in legally instead; that change in itself promotes assimilation, by giving immigrants more of a permanent stake in their new lives here.

The expansion of legal immigration is also supported by security considerations. The most basic functions of government—those concerning national defense as well as the domestic protection of persons and property—demand that we have the ability to screen immigrants before entry, to find and deport those who commit crimes while here, and to prevent those who mean us harm from entering in the first place if we can. One of the major reasons to liberalize *legal* immigration is that it would make it *unnecessary* for people to sneak across the border for honorable purposes—and therefore we could reasonably assume that anyone who came here illegally would probably be up to no good.

Government may be able to do one more thing to encourage legal immigration while reducing illegal immigration: limit "birthright" citizenship to those whose parents are in the country legally. The 14th amendment to the Constitution extends citizenship to "[a]ll persons born or naturalized in the United States, *and subject to the jurisdiction thereof.*" The Supreme Court has rejected the claim that the italicized language excludes the children of illegal immigrants, but Congress arguably has the authority under section 5 of the 14th amendment to pass remedial legislation reversing that interpretation. At the very least Congress should try.

Other governmental solutions that have been proposed to "secure our borders" seem far less promising. For example, it's hard to believe that a wall or fence along our southern border is practical, or that its benefits could be justified by its cost. First, it's a *very* long border to police. Second, it's only *one* border, so to the extent that we're building a wall or fence for security reasons, it doesn't even pretend to be a complete solution. Third, as many as half of all illegal immigrants come here legally on student, work, or tourist visas which they then overstay; no physical barrier will do anything about that half of the problem. In all these respects, closing the border to illegal immigrants would be as hard as closing the border to illegal drugs, and we have already wasted tens of billions of dollars in that attempt.

Similarly, the idea of heavier regulation or tougher penalties for employers will simply impose more unfair burdens on small businesses, for whom the burdens of regulatory compliance are already heavier than for large businesses. Many tout the advantages of the "E-Verify" program for checking work authorizations online. That may be fine for businesses large enough to have full-time human resources personnel. But for small businesses where the owner does the hiring and firing, E-Verify is just one more government requirement to comply with and one more way to get sued by a job applicant or investigated by the federal government. We should let business owners run their businesses instead of essentially drafting them to serve without pay as immigration cops.

What about the illegal immigrants who are already here? To be just, our policy should not reward those who broke the law to get here; should not grant them amnesty nor allow them to "cut the line" in front of others who have waited far too long already to immigrate here legally. But to be compassionate, our policy should recognize that the vast majority of illegal immigrants have come here only to live in peace with their neighbors and make life better for themselves and their families; most would be model citizens if citizenship were open to them.

Furthermore, to be practical, our policy should recognize that finding and deporting many millions of people who don't want to be found or deported is very costly ($12,500 per deportee in 2011), and not very effective (fewer than 400,000 were deported in 2011, or less than 4% of the estimated number of illegal aliens here—and 2011 saw the most deportations on record). We should still make the effort with respect to people who are committing crimes of violence, but the expense just isn't justified for people who are actually contributing positively to their communities here. Remember: immigration of peaceful, productive people is good for us.

These countervailing considerations suggest that we must find a way to assimilate the millions of people who are currently here illegally. It is increasingly difficult to discuss this rationally, because words like "amnesty," "self-deportation," and "path to citizenship" have already been poisoned in various communities, and now tend to generate more heat than light. With no perfect solutions and valid points on both sides, this ought to be a subject on which compromise is not only excusable but essential. We might permit illegal immigrants to apply for work visas or permanent residency on terms that (a) are no more favorable in any respect than those available to new immigrants, (b) require proof of the payment of taxes (or back-taxes) for the entire period of their illegal residence; and (c) take some account of the extent to which they applicants have already integrated themselves into our society. (For example, have they been continuously employed? Have they become proficient in English?) But there is nothing uniquely reasonable about these suggestions, and the goal of legislative action here should be a successful compromise, not a roof-raising campaign speech.

Readers who find these conclusions discouraging might wish to reflect on why it's so hard for the government to keep immigrants out of the United States. It's hard because the desire to come here is so strong. And the desire is strong precisely because this has been, for the last two centuries, the place above all others on Earth where liberty has been the central social good binding the community together. It is easy to understand the impulse to protect that liberty from the uncertainties created by a huge influx of "outsiders." But it would be tragic, here as in other areas, for us to "protect" our liberty right out of existence, by building walls, requiring paperwork for everyday life, and exercising sweeping police powers to enforce restrictive laws. Perhaps, in the end, the only way to make our liberty truly secure is to allow others to share it.

Reforming Congress

*We desperately need to dismantle
the incumbency-protection machine.*

When I ran for Congress in 2010, only 21% of registered voters approved of the job Congress was doing. Nonetheless, I predicted that at least three-quarters of the incumbent House members would be re-elected that fall. The actual number? 85%. And that was actually quite low in historical terms. The re-election rate had been above 94% in the seven preceding elections, and above 98% in three of those seven elections. In fact, the re-election rate had only fallen below 90% *twice* in the preceding *forty years.*

How can this possibly happen? Because no matter how they argue, incumbent Democrats and incumbent Republicans have formed a bipartisan consensus that Congressional seats should be held by career politicians who are re-elected easily no matter what.

This is not what the framers of our Constitution intended, but it is also not new. Around 1910, the famous Tammany Hall politician George Washington Plunkitt expressed what I take to be the dominant view:

> On election day I try to pile up as big a majority as I can against George Wanmaker, the Republican leader of the Fifteenth. Any other day George and I are the best of friends. I can go to him and say: "George, I want you to place this friend of mine." He says: "All right, Senator." Or vice versa.
>
> You see, we differ on tariffs and currencies and all them things, but *we agree on the main proposition that when a man works in politics, he should get something out of it.*
> [from "Plunkitt of Tammany Hall"]

We are on notice, then, that incumbents tend to agree that political deals favoring insiders are perfectly legitimate, even desirable. We need to counteract this attitude of entitlement. Here are three suggestions.

Term limits

Republicans promised us term limits in 1994, but somehow they became less interested once they had captured a majority of the House. Here's why we should embrace the cause of term limits once again.

First, term limits reduce our legislators' dependence on special interests by reducing their own "need" for re-election. Normal people try not to get fired in the middle of a promising career, and career politicians behave pretty much the same way. The primary reason we need term limits is not because our current representatives are bad people; it is because they are ordinary people and our current system creates unhealthy incentives for these ordinary people to try to hang onto their offices as long as possible.

Second, term limits will tend to make Congress look a lot more like the citizens it governs. If a stint in Congress were seen as short-term service to one's country rather than a long-term career path, then representatives would be more likely to have recent experience as workers, business owners, parents, taxpayers, etc. The careerism that is currently rampant in our Congress robs us of this diversity and leaves in its stead a deplorable sameness. The lack of imagination that this spawns is only compounded by the fact that the turnover is so low. Not only do we get careerists playing it safe year after year; we get the *same* careerists playing it safe year after year.

Third, term limits will tend to discourage disreputable conduct, by shuffling the deck often enough to prevent excessive coziness. It would be naïve to think that term limits would stop lobbyists from trying to cultivate "friends in high places," but more frequent turnover will make it harder for a representative to become completely captive.

Some claim term limits would give agency bureaucrats and Congressional staffers too much power because the federal government is too complicated for an inexperienced member of Congress to understand. This criticism reverses cause and effect. Our government is certainly too complicated, but perhaps the best way to uncomplicate it is to subject it to the scrutiny of many fresh eyes in each Congress.

Redistricting reform

Most congressional districts are now gerrymandered to produce a predictable result. Politicians have always done this—the word "gerrymander" goes back to the 1790s—but the dramatic improvements in computing power over the last few decades have made it possible to fix elections with certainty. This is terrible for self-government.

The worst effect of gerrymandering is the most obvious one: It lets politicians choose their voters instead of the other way around. In Maryland's 8th District, Republican Connie Morella had been elected to eight straight terms before the Democrats in Annapolis decided to change the district boundaries to give Democrats a heavy majority. At the next election, *voila!* The new representative was Democrat Chris Van Hollen. And he won every successive election with those district lines. This year, the lines have changed again, because the Democrats in Annapolis decided they wanted to win seven of Maryland's eight House seats instead of just six. Could there be anything more unseemly? Or more corrosive of our political institutions?

Gerrymandering discourages minority populations from voting at all, because they quickly learn that unless the party bosses drew their district in such a way as to put them in a semi-permanent majority, it really doesn't matter whether they vote or not. Predictably, they increasingly decide to skip it.

Democrats in Annapolis have gerrymandered Maryland so aggressively that some representatives don't seem to represent any real community at all. In the 2010 election, there were no community organizations in Maryland's 2nd District who were willing to schedule a debate among the candidates for the House seat held by C.A. "Dutch" Ruppersberger. That's because debate-hosting groups like the League of Women Voters are normally organized by city or county, and there was no city or county that was even mostly in Maryland's 2nd District. Instead, the district was cobbled together from relatively small pieces of four different political subdivisions. As a result, no community organization considered Mr. Ruppersberger to be "their" congressman during the election season. He's the congressman from nowhere.

I'm convinced that gerrymandering also lowers the quality of the people we bring to Congress, by rewarding predictable conformity to the party line over thoughtfulness and candor. Consider the case of Rep. Danny K. Davis (D - IL), who in 2003 *carried a crown to Rev. Sun Myung Moon on a pillow during a private coronation ceremony in the Capitol!* (Moon then declared himself the Messiah and stated that his teachings had helped Hitler and Stalin be reborn.) When I first read that astonishing story, I looked up Davis's margin of victory in the 2002 election and was not the least bit surprised to find that he had collected a robust 83.2% of the votes in his district. Only a person in a *very* safe district can afford to use such poor judgment.

Many people believe that redistricting cannot be reformed because line-drawing exercises are inherently subjective. This is actually not true. Some very clever people at rangevoting.org tout something called the "shortest splitline algorithm," which uses geometry and population density to draw districts according to stable and pre-existing rules that cannot be manipulated by politicians. Interestingly, the site includes Maryland's (2002) congressional districts in a list of egregiously gerrymandered districts. Their comment on the redistricting job that gave Chris Van Hollen his seat? "Holy sea of rattlesnakes Batman! *Numerous* go out to sea and come back to land districts, *amazingly* squirrelly boundary shapes."

Unfortunately, we cannot expect any reform of this extremely undemocratic institution from the people who owe their election to it. To cure the plague of gerrymandering, we first need to win at the ballot box even with the deck stacked against us.

Fundamental tax reform

This may be the most important reform of all. The Internal Revenue Code, weighing in at a hefty 5.5 million words, is an affront to human rationality. Its complexity saps *billions* of hours of productive energy from the economy and provides an all-too-tempting hiding place for political favors to well-connected special interests.

In addition, the dizzying welter of rates, exemptions, deductions, and credits has undermined social consensus about who should pay what. High-income Americans sometimes argue that they are paying more than their fair share. For example, the Census Bureau reports that in 2000 the richest 20% of households earned 49.65% of the income but paid 76.6% of the taxes. Is that fair? The middle fifth earned 14.85% of the income but paid only 6.9% of the taxes. Is that fair? Meanwhile, lower- and middle-income taxpayers complain that the rich have too many ways to shield their income from taxation. Wages for a hard day's labor are subject not only to income tax but to the regressive payroll (social security) tax, while dividends and capital gains enjoy preferential income tax rates and are not subject to payroll tax at all. Is that fair? And if the rich really think the poor have it too soft, why don't they just quit their desk jobs and earn less? The subjectivity inherent in the fairness question makes it a perennial occasion for class warfare.

Better alternatives abound, including the Flat Tax, the FairTax, and the intriguing "Automated Payment Transaction Tax." Any of these proposals would be preferable to our current income tax, provided that the income tax is eliminated. Simply layering another tax on top of the existing income tax (as many believe the Obama administration will propose with a "Value Added Tax") would be a disaster.

Tax policy is usually considered primarily as a matter of economic regulation, but we should also consider it as a matter of political philosophy. In particular, a flat tax, sales tax, or APT tax would emphasize our common membership in one community and our common responsibility to ensure that public needs are paid for. For example, if we were already paying a retail sales tax of 25% and we decided to spend $550 billion for a prescription drug benefit, we could either raise the sales tax, cut spending elsewhere, or borrow the money. The one thing we would not be able to do would be to start a big fight about whether the cost of the benefit should somehow be borne by some of our citizens and not others. Even though the rich would pay more tax than the poor, every citizen would be subject to that same 25% rate, and would have a clear stake in the spending decisions we face as a nation. That's a lot of citizenship and a lot of community at a very reasonable price, and we save 6.4 billion hours in the bargain.

Trusting the States

*Congress should not legislate on any subject
the states can handle.*

Perhaps the most important innovation the founders incorpo-
rated into our Constitution was the notion of a government
limited strictly to a list of enumerated powers. Naturally, the
list emphasized subjects that were bigger than any one state,
like national defense, interstate commerce, and naturalization
of citizens. The individual states were to remain sovereign as
to everything else. Today we might put air transportation and
telecommunications regulation in the same category. But job
training? Elementary school funding? Drug laws? Health
care? Abortion? Nothing about these issues requires uniform
national policy in every state.

There are at least three very pragmatic reasons to prefer state
and local government solutions to federal government solutions.
First, when it comes to solving social problems in a country as
large and diverse as the United States, one size definitely does

not fit all. A 55-mph speed limit made a great deal more sense along the densely populated Eastern seaboard than it ever made for people driving between Reno and Salt Lake City.

Second, even where the states are similarly situated, a diversity of policy approaches permits us to develop experience with different potential solutions so that all the nation's eggs need not be placed in any one basket. When states pursue different solutions simultaneously, the most successful pave the way for others to gravitate toward what works.

Third, even where each state takes essentially the same approach to essentially the same problem, smaller programs closer to the people typically have greater responsiveness, accountability, and effectiveness. Local citizens and officials are usually better acquainted with local facts, and money that comes directly from the local community is almost always spent more carefully than money that comes from Washington.

Furthermore, simply as an element of political freedom, different states should be free to assign different relative priorities to issues. For example, one state may choose higher taxes and more generous social services while another chooses lower taxes and less generous government services. If "to govern is to choose," this is a basic function of self-government. Citizens of different states may just differ on fundamental issues of principle. Unless the difference itself constitutes a national problem, we should let them differ.

It is strange but true that some of the most divisive issues in national politics are issues that do not require national solutions at all. We can use the abortion issue—almost certainly the most divisive political issue of the last forty years—to illustrate the point. The legality of artificial abortion was being hashed out state by state in the 1960s, but activists on both sides found that unsatisfactory. Many people who lost the debate in their home states were eager for a second chance at the national level, and many people who won in their home states were eager to extend their victory to other states regardless of what the people in those states thought. Unfortunately, the Supreme Court nationalized the issue in *Roe v. Wade* (1973), and from that day to the present it has been a key "wedge" issue in every national election. It will almost certainly remain divisive as long as we foolishly persist in trying to address it on a national level.

Here are a few of the issues (in addition to abortion) that Congresses and Presidents have unwisely turned into federal issues:

- *Education*. Believe me, I understand the view that our schools are letting us down. After all, for twelve years now, most members of Congress have apparently been so lousy at math that they are unable to tell the difference between positive and negative numbers at budget time. But a top-down, one-size-fits-all model of education is unlikely to help. I have two children, and I don't even send them to the same schools, because they're different and they need different things. It's ironic that educators nearly all extol the virtues of diversity when they are talking about the composition of the student body at a given school, but fail to recognize the value of diversity in the education itself. The top-down approach is bad for students, and it would be wise to get rid of it *even if it were free*—but of course it's actually terribly expensive. The federal government should exit the field of education as quickly as possible.

- *Drug prohibition*. Drug use may often be self-destructive, like alcohol consumption. But states should only regulate the effect of drug use on other people, as they do with alcohol consumption. I believe our experience shows that total prohibition is *not* possible (we can't even keep drugs out of prison!), and that the attempt to make prohibition work has caused much more harm to society (violent crime, high rates of incarceration for non-violent offenders) than legal drug use would cause. But even apart from those considerations, I still see little reason for drug policy to be decided at the federal level. In fact, I do not see any provision in the U.S. Constitution which, properly interpreted, would authorize the federal government to override a state's judgment about what substances an individual can consume.

• *Same-sex marriage*. Most of the people on both sides of the "same-sex marriage" issue share the (usually unexamined) belief that government needs to regulate marriage in order for it to survive as an institution. But our closest legal cousins in England and Wales managed to do without any state regulation of marriage until 1754. The reason we have a tradition of government regulation in this country is because the Pilgrims (having been religious dissenters who could not obtain the sacrament of marriage from the Church of England) liked the *Dutch* practice of making marriage civil rather than religious. It's time to privatize marriage. "Common law" marriages (no license, no ceremony) have been recognized in the majority of U.S. jurisdictions at one time or another and are still valid today in eleven states and the District of Columbia. In light of this historical record, the case for state regulation of marriage is pretty weak. The case for *federal* regulation is weaker still. This is simply none of Congress's business.

Does the reader, by any chance, notice anything these four issues have in common? If you said, "They really fire up the base on both sides of the aisle," move to the head of the class. It would be unjust to claim that *all* politicians at the federal level are consciously exploiting these issues for their own personal gain; each issue is pushed at the federal level by people who believe very strongly that they are working to improve society. But it is perfectly fair to observe that these issues cast a long shadow across the federal electoral landscape, dimming the light available for seeing other issues clearly.

Perhaps more to the point, the attempt to impose centralized, one-size-fits-all solutions from Washington deprives us all of the advances that usually come from allowing states (and individuals!) to try many different approaches to a given problem. At a time when the people in Congress can't even balance a budget, do we really want them to spend more time on social engineering? Are they really the people we want to put in charge of molding the national character?

PART II:

Selected Lessays

On the Importance of Political Persuasion

I was a first-time candidate in 2010, and I learned some surprising things.

- I learned that running for Congress can be extremely embarrassing, particularly for those of us who hold Congress in the lowest possible regard right now.

- I learned that answering voters' questions with answers that are short, complete, articulate, and persuasive is harder than it looks.

- I learned that the relentless gerrymandering in which both major parties engage has corrupted the electoral process much more than I had suspected.

- I learned that the greatest—indeed, almost the only—opportunities for debate and voter outreach are provided by organizations whose members are more or less committed to one party or the other.

- And I learned that people who are completely alienated from the electoral process—who aren't registered, or don't vote—are nearly impossible to entice back into the system.

But the most important thing I learned is this: Campaigns are just as important as elections. At first blush, this is a surprising claim, because candidates and their supporters generally speak as if everything depends on Election Day. But my experience has been that voters who attend campaign events are not just trying to learn which candidate matches up best with views the voters already hold. Attentive voters also use campaigns as an opportunity to question their own views; to think about new issues, or perhaps to think about old issues in new ways or in the light of new facts. In the long run, it's the social consensus that emerges from this give and take that *really* determines what happens after Election Day, no matter which candidate wins the election.

If we want to get our country back on the right track, we need to renew and sustain a strong political consensus that consistently favors personal liberty over government power, regardless of whether we're talking about entitlement spending, economic regulations, civil liberties, or foreign policy.

If you think that renewing and sustaining a strong political consensus sounds harder than winning an election—well, that's the way it sounds to me too. For my part, it means that I can't just cobble together a few positions that poll well and call it a day, as establishment candidates do. I also need to *persuade* voters who don't already agree with me about the overall soundness of a small-government worldview. I need to persuade voters—in Maryland, mostly Democratic voters—that we can have a much brighter future if we cut our government down to size and dispense once and for all with the illusion that government is capable of giving us everything we want.

My campaign essays are an attempt to do just that: to reach out to voters who are frankly skeptical of Libertarian arguments (or in some cases, the caricatures of those arguments) and make the case for personal liberty as forcefully as I can. I will try at all times to carry on the debate with civility, and I hope anyone who carries these discussions further will do the same.

But you, dear reader, must do your part as well. It is not enough for you to read my essays, not enough even to reward me with your vote. You also need to help spread our message to your friends and neighbors. Encourage them to read the essays you find convincing. Mention the Libertarian alternative in your political discussions. Join some of the social networks from where Libertarian news and commentary circulate, and invite your friends to do the same. Write letters to the editor of your favorite paper. Get involved. Together, "less we can."

What Do Libertarians Stand for?

When I first ran for Congress in 2010, some of the people in my audiences had never met a Libertarian and had little or no idea what positions Libertarians take in modern politics. Fortunately, libertarianism has been growing rapidly in popularity recently, and today there are so many excellent introductions to libertarianism that it's hard to recommend just a few.

For over 25 years, the Advocates for Self Government (www.theadvocates.com) have published books, pamphlets, and now electronic media to educate people about libertarianism. Here is one of their most concise summaries:

> Libertarians support maximum liberty in both personal and economic matters. They advocate a much smaller government; one that is limited to protecting individuals from coercion and violence. Libertarians tend to embrace individual responsibility, oppose government bureaucracy and taxes, promote private charity, tolerate diverse lifestyles, support the free market, and defend civil liberties.

Elsewhere, the Advocates note that "[t]he core idea is simply stated, but profound and far-reaching in its implications":

> Libertarianism is thus the combination of liberty (the freedom to live your life in any peaceful way you choose), responsibility (the prohibition against the use of force against others, except in defense), and tolerance (honoring and respecting the peaceful choices of others).

For another perspective, let's look at a website that didn't exist in 2010, the exemplary Libertarianism.org:

> Libertarianism is the belief that each person has the right to live his life as he chooses so long as he respects the equal rights of others. Libertarians defend each person's right to life, liberty, and property. . . . Force should be reserved for prohibiting or punishing those who themselves use force, such as murderers, robbers, rapists, kidnappers, and defrauders (who practice a kind of theft).

The focus on equality here is crucial. Libertarians think each citizen's right to pursue his own happiness without government interference is limited only by the equal rights of others. Governments today violate that basic equality not just through overtly discriminatory actions (like the federal ban on same-sex marriage), but also through many seemingly arcane economic policies that may even appear non-coercive at first blush. Tax credits for Prius owners force some people to subsidize others' car preferences. Bailouts in the banking and auto industries force taxpayers to pay for other people's failures and deny well-managed competitors of the bailed-out firms their just rewards for prudently managing their own affairs. Libertarians oppose this Santa Claus mentality not because they hate free stuff, but because they know the stuff is not free and they don't think it should be taken from others by force.

The writers at Libertarianism.org continue:

> Most people live their own lives by that code of ethics. Libertarians believe that that code should be applied consistently, even to the actions of governments, which should be restricted to protecting people from violations of their rights. Governments should not use their powers to censor speech, conscript the young, prohibit voluntary exchanges, steal or "redistribute" property, or interfere in the lives of individuals who are otherwise minding their own business.

As this paragraph makes clear, libertarianism is *essentially political*. In other words, libertarianism speaks to the proper relationship between the state and the individual; it does not speak to what individuals ought morally to do voluntarily. Thus, to take an obvious example, Libertarians overwhelmingly oppose the nation's "war on drugs" even though we may tell our own kids they'll be grounded for life if we catch them with pot.

Some people wonder why Libertarians draw such a sharp distinction between proper conduct for governments and proper conduct for individuals. As we have already seen, the political equality of all citizens is perhaps the most important philosophical reason. But there are many other practical reasons for insisting on a very narrow scope for government action. Libertarians believe that when government fails to confine itself to the protection of persons and property, its actions are generally unnecessary, routinely inferior to private action, and very frequently counterproductive. We'll have an opportunity to look at some of the reasons for this throughout the rest of this book.

Are you a Libertarian?

The Libertarian Party is our nation's third-largest political party, but that's not a reason to join. (Of course, it's not a reason *not* to join, either.) The only good reason to join the Libertarian Party is to support political principles that appeal to your reason and your conscience.

The Advocates for Self Government have (again, for many years) published a ten-question quiz designed to help people measure the degree to which they accept libertarian principles. Here are the ten questions, each to be answered with a Yes, a No, or a Maybe:

1. Government should not censor speech, press, media, or internet.

2. Military service should be voluntary. There should be no draft.

3. There should be no laws regarding sex for consenting adults.

4. Repeal laws prohibiting adult possession and use of drugs.

5. There should be no National ID card.

6. End "corporate welfare." No government handouts to business.

7. End government barriers to international free trade.

8. Let people control their own retirement; privatize Social Security.

9. Replace government welfare with private charity.

10. Cut taxes and government spending by 50% or more.

(If you want to take the quiz and find out how libertarian you are, go to www.theadvocates.org/quiz.)

If you begin to suspect that you just might be a Libertarian don't be too surprised. More and more Democrats, Republicans, Greens, and independents have figured out that the "usual suspects" in the two major parties have no earthly idea what's ailing our society or how we can return to peace and prosperity. The leaders of these parties—people who have attained "leadership" status largely by hanging around too long—suffer from an idea deficit that is every bit as daunting as our budget deficit. As a result, the sclerotic parties they lead are on the brink of intellectual bankruptcy themselves. And once you've seen through the incumbents' shtick, it's nearly impossible to keep supporting them. Fortunately, you don't have to; you can join the Libertarian Party instead.

But you don't have to join the Libertarian Party to understand that, right now, libertarian principles provide our best hope of reining in our government and restoring peace and prosperity. And you don't have to think the Libertarian Party is right about every conceivable hypothetical question to know that it's right about the things that need the most urgent attention in 2012. Voting Libertarian sends the unambiguous message that our national government is too big, too dumb, and too expensive. Send that message. Vote Libertarian.

Further reading

At the top of the list is David Boaz's excellent introduction, *Libertarianism: A Primer.* This book surveys both the political and economic foundations of libertarianism, concisely and powerfully.

Boaz's book was first published in 1997, and for that reason it makes a nice contrast with Ron Paul's 2008 contribution, *Revolution: A Manifesto*. Dr. Paul's central thesis in this book (as elsewhere) is that we have departed from the principles of our nation's founding in ways that systematically make us less free. It's a great explanation of why we were on the wrong course long before the financial crisis of 2008 and long before President Obama took over. Dr. Paul published a more issue-oriented treatment in 2011, *Liberty Defined: 50 Essential Issues that Affect Our Freedom*. It's also excellent.

Readers who are mostly interested in the economic case for smaller government will enjoy Henry Hazlitt's 1946 classic, *Economics in One Lesson*. Hazlitt draws out the implications of one of the simplest and most important ideas in political economy, namely the fact that government largesse always involves tradeoffs and that it is important to pay attention not just to the things politicians promise to give us, but to the things we will not be able to provide for ourselves if we let them use private resources for their bright ideas.

Finally, if you want to read a prescient primary work by a Nobel laureate and prominent libertarian scholar (though he hated the word "libertarian" and preferred to call himself a "classical liberal"), try *The Road to Serfdom* by F.A. Hayek. Hayek, an Austrian who experienced Europe's descent into fascism firsthand, published this book in 1944 to connect the dots primarily for British readers who did not understand the way that centralized economic planning systematically tends toward the suppression of political freedom.

Ice, Wind, and Freedom

My deodorant says on the label that it "smells like ice, wind, and freedom." Now you and I know that my deodorant doesn't actually smell like freedom; marketing people just use the language of freedom to sell their deodorant, because freedom is popular. It's pure puffery, and it means nothing because we all know that *no* deodorant smells like freedom. The "freedom" talk is just a harmless gimmick.

Unfortunately, sometimes the same marketing method is used not to sell products, but to sell candidates. And that's anything but harmless, because candidates really differ quite a bit on their fundamental attitudes toward freedom: its importance, its limits, and even its definition. Democrats and Republicans alike use the *language* of freedom to make you cast your vote for one of them. Sometimes their candidates talk so much about freedom that they almost sound Libertarian. Some promise to free you from endless foreign wars; or to free you from job-killing regulations; or to free you from the power of large corporations; or to free you from government intrusion in your personal affairs.

Do they deliver more freedom? No; no more than my deodorant. But they keep making the same promises. Why? Because we keep letting them fool us.

Fortunately, more and more voters have seen through the phony promises. Increasingly, they've noticed that only the Libertarian Party actually proposes to free us from all the ways modern government intrudes on our lives—to free us from more bombings overseas, as well as more bailouts and Big-Brotherism here at home.

So to stop you from voting for what you really want, the Democrats and Republicans tell you that you'll be "wasting your vote" if you vote Libertarian. They want you to vote for the lesser of two evils.

This is just another gimmick, and before you fall for it please ask yourself: Is there any other important decision you make that way? Did you marry the lesser of two evils? Would anyone suggest that you worship the lesser of two evils in order to go along with the rest of the crowd? How many of you wish you had to live in one of two houses that someone else offered you? How many of you make yourselves buy one of the two most popular cars instead of the one you really want? It's *your vote*. Don't give it away to a candidate who doesn't reflect your idea of good government.

If you're still on the fence about this, I encourage you to think back over the last two or three votes you've cast in national elections. If you're *glad* you voted for Barack Obama, or John McCain, fine. If you wish you could buy *another* John Kerry or George W. Bush bumper sticker to put on your *next* car, then by all means keep voting Republican or Democrat.

But if you now look back on any of those votes with regret; if you're now haunted by the feeling that *you asked for* some of the trouble in which we now find ourselves; *that* was a wasted vote. That vote didn't smell like freedom. That vote stank.

The good news is: It's a new year, and you get another chance to vote for what you really want. If you value liberty, vote Libertarian.

Thinking Small

With public approval of Congress touching all-time lows, why do we keep electing the same people to give us the same kind of government we already don't like? Gerrymandering is surely part of the answer, especially in Maryland. But we also need to sharpen our thinking about how government works, and why it fails. Here are seven things we need to learn (or perhaps remember) if we want better government.

1. Government can't solve every problem. In real life, there are always more problems in any society; we never run out. If we expect government to solve them all, we'll always need new government programs—including new programs to fix the old programs. This is a key reason why government expands in good times and bad. People who want less government cannot keep asking government to do more. We won't have smaller government until we stop looking to government for all the answers.

2. You can't solve real problems with ideal solutions. Solutions to real-life problems have to work in real life, but we often debate policy issues as if new government programs will work exactly as we intend. Wrong. Experience tells us they will be flawed in both design and implementation. They will cost more than we expect and do less than we hope. People will try to avoid rules they don't like. There will often be unintended consequences. So when somebody says "there oughtta be a law" about something, we need to factor in those real-life downsides.

3. Power doesn't make people smarter or more virtuous. Candidates almost always say they respect the wisdom of the voters. So why don't they trust us to choose our own light bulbs? Why do they make people get licenses to cut hair? Why don't they trust us to decide how tall our shrubberies should be? Ultimately, most government programs assume that government officials are either smarter or more attuned to the public good than ordinary citizens are. But the people regulating light bulbs, barbershops, and shrubberies—and banks, and airline security, and so on – are mostly the same as the people we see in the supermarket. Some are very smart, and most mean well—but they're all fallible. We shouldn't imagine these same people will run our lives any better just because we give them power. If anything, power tends to make people worse.

4. Power attracts influence. With any government program, the people who have the most to gain or lose spend a lot of time and money on influence—a whole lot more time and money than ordinary citizens do. Even without actual corruption, the people who have the most direct interests will inevitably have better information and better access than the public at large, so their voices will dominate the debate. Over time, then, government regulation is more likely to protect powerful economic interests than to constrain them. Expanding government power simply gives the already-powerful another lever to pull.

5. Power magnifies mistakes. Everybody makes mistakes, public and private sectors alike. But government mistakes are bigger because they affect all of us. And this problem only gets worse as the government gets bigger. A mistake by a town council affects a whole town, but no one else. A mistake at the federal level affects the entire country. Minimizing the damage done by dumb ideas is a good reason to keep government as close to the people as possible.

6. Power uses failure to justify expansion. When is the last time you heard a government program head say his agency wasn't achieving its mission and should therefore be discontinued? Instead, government officials nearly always tell us the solution to bad government is more government. They tend to ask for (or give themselves) more money, more power, or both. We need to start viewing these requests for government expansion as confessions of failure. When a school chief tells us his school can't educate children adequately for $20,000 per pupil, he ought to be telling us that in a resignation letter.

7. The clown show isn't over until the clowns are gone. If most of the foregoing seems obvious, why don't elected officials seem to know it? Because we don't vote as if we've learned the lessons ourselves. We keep electing people who think they can improve society by using the force of law (backed by real guns, courts, and jails) to take decisions away from individuals and centralize them in Washington, in state capitals, and in county seats. Until we start doing something different in the voting booth, we run the risk indicated by a Chinese proverb: If we don't change direction, we will end up where we're headed.

We have every reason to be dissatisfied with government right now. But we'll never fix the problems without recognizing that they originate in our own mistaken attitudes toward the proper role of government in society.

Libertarians on the Political Spectrum?

People in an unfamiliar neighborhood often look to surroundings for clues as to whether they feel (or should feel) comfortable. That's the spirit, I think, in which some people who read my description of Libertarianism follow up by asking where Libertarianism fits along the so-called "political spectrum" that is typically used to describe Democrats and Republicans.

The short answer—the answer that plays along with the idea that there is such a thing as a one-dimensional "political spectrum"—is that Libertarians hold many positions that journalists would place to the "left" of the Democrats, and many other positions that journalists would place to the "right" of the Republicans.

For example, Libertarians want to end the war on drugs. We want to rein in presidential power to commit us to undeclared wars. We stand up for civil liberties that have been violated in the name of the "war on terror." In newspaper-speak, these positions are "left" of the Democrats, at least in practice. Consequently, many voters who think of themselves as Democrats but who are dissatisfied with their supine representatives in Congress should give the Libertarians a careful look.

At the same time, however, Libertarians oppose government interference with free markets, including many kinds of interference supported by Republicans in recent years. We oppose not just Obamacare but also the Bush expansion of Medicare entitlements. We oppose not just the Obama stimulus and bailout legislation of early 2009 but also the Bush stimulus and bailout legislation of early and late 2008. We favor the wholesale elimination of federal programs in areas like agriculture and energy that should be handled by private markets. In newspaper-speak, these positions are to the "right" of the Republicans, and many voters who think of themselves as Republicans could send a much clearer message about their preference for smaller government if they were to vote Libertarian.

The main reason Libertarian positions don't fall neatly along a left-right "spectrum" is because Libertarians apply a consistent philosophy of maximizing personal liberty, not only in economics but wherever civil liberties are concerned. By contrast, Democrats and Republicans take inconsistent positions about the extent to which government should interfere with personal liberty. Democrats make a big show of staying out of your bedroom, but they tend to micromanage the way you earn a living, tax you heavily on whatever you earn, and place massive bureaucracies in charge of fundamentally personal issues like medical care and retirement. Republicans claim to be pro-business, but in practice they express this by giving tax breaks to special interests instead of simply staying out of the way and letting markets work. And despite the way Republicans disparage federal bureaucracy on the campaign trail, they seem all too happy to treat government as practically omniscient when it is accusing people of crimes, operating "no fly" lists, or deciding who should rule Iraq or Libya.

For better or worse, then, the left-to-right "spectrum" metaphor isn't a very useful guide to contemporary American politics because there is no single political value according to which the positions of Democrats and Republicans can be compared in a straight line from left to right. It would be more helpful to say that Libertarians consistently oppose interference with personal liberty, whereas Democrats and Republicans often favor large, powerful, and intrusive government at the expense of personal liberty, albeit in different areas. Anyone who is consistently in favor of smaller government and greater personal liberty should be voting Libertarian.

How Liberty Creates Prosperity

Most people in the United States take for granted that free-market economies "work" better than centrally planned economies. That is, almost everyone in any domestic political debate will agree, without thinking about it much, that placing the government in charge of how many shoes get made, and what the price of corn should be, and where we all work, would be disastrous for everyone. We've seen other countries try it, and we know it doesn't work.

It's good that we don't have to argue about this. But an unfortunate side-effect of *not* arguing is that many voters don't really understand *why* free-market economies are more prosperous, or *why* government interference usually makes us poorer even when it falls well short of total centralization. And that makes these voters suckers for politicians who promise to "improve" unpopular economic outcomes like high gas prices or electricity brownouts. So let's look in very basic terms at how liberty creates prosperity.

Economic reporting often focuses on arcane aggregate statistics of dubious reliability and uncertain meaning, so it's important to emphasize that economics is about how to solve the very real and very human problem of how to feed, clothe, and shelter ourselves. Humans have material needs, as well as a natural drive to satisfy those needs. We also have a natural inclination to satisfy our needs with as little effort as possible. The overriding goal of all economic activity is really only this: to satisfy human needs as abundantly as possible with the minimum amount of work.

One of the principal ways we generate abundance is by trading with each other. Why? Because we don't all have the same skills or aptitudes, and once we get beyond the most basic necessities we don't all have the same tastes and desires either. Trading allows us to specialize; to focus our work on what we like and what we're good at, and trade for the other stuff we need. If one neighbor just builds houses and the other just grows food, both families end up warmer and better fed. That's why most of us are better off buying hamburger from the butcher instead of raising our own steer. It's also why it's a mistake to think of free markets as essentially "**selfish.**" One of the miracles of the free market is that it facilitates very sophisticated forms of social cooperation among people who aren't getting explicit directions from anyone and who may not even know of each other's existence.

In theory, people could trade without ever using money. The wheat farmer could pay the blacksmith in wheat, and the carpenter could demand fish for building the fisherman's house. But money makes trades much easier. Money allows fishermen to buy houses even from carpenters who hate fish, and it allows farmers to sell wheat to blacksmiths and carpenters and fishermen alike without calculating separate rates of exchange with each. Instead, people with goods or services to sell can reduce their terms of exchange to a single price in money. That's true whether the money in question is paper, gold, stones, or wampum.

When we're allowed to engage in purely voluntary trades with each other, something fascinating happens. We benefit not only from the exchanges themselves, but from the price signals that emerge from those exchanges. The prices allow us to fine-tune the relative amounts of work we put into buying and selling different goods and services. When the price of potatoes rises, people with the ability to produce potatoes try to supply more of them and people who eat potatoes try to eat fewer. Not everyone will become a potato grower, and not everyone will stop eating potatoes, but some people will act on the signals sent by the rising price, and that will tend to counteract the price increase and bring demand and supply back into balance. It is this highly decentralized process of continuous adjustment that in fact guides consumption, production, and investment in free economies.

Our ancestors learned to work, to trade, to use money, and to respond to price signals, all without government direction. In fact, anthropologists have evidence that we were engaged in trade (and the specialization of labor) as long as 100,000 years ago, long before we had anything like the modern state. Government can help, to be sure: by clearly defining property rights, and by protecting people from violence, theft, fraud, and broken promises.

But unfortunately, modern governments often want to do more. When the price signals from free trade deliver bad news (*e.g., we have too many houses and not enough oil*), politicians motivated by personal ambition have an incentive to try to "help" us by "correcting" unpleasant market outcomes. Fortunately, we can now see at least some of the ways government interference makes us worse off.

First, government makes us worse off by compelling or prohibiting voluntary trades. If Jones would like to trade some of his fish for some of Smith's wheat, and Smith is equally willing, we can be sure that the trade makes both Smith and Jones better off (by their own lights, at least). That's not true if Jones is *forced* to sell fish or Smith is *forced* to sell wheat (or if either is forced to buy health insurance). Indeed, a forced exchange of wheat for fish almost certainly makes either Smith or Jones worse off, because if the trade were mutually advantageous there would be no need to force the two sides into it. And government usually makes *both* Smith and Jones worse off when it *prohibits* them from trading even though they would prefer to do so.

Second, government makes almost everyone worse off when it fiddles with prices, because that distorts our allocation of society's resources. We may not like high gas prices, but they tell us something important about gasoline, namely that it is getting scarcer and that we would be well advised to take actions that increase production, reduce consumption, or both. Capping prices would hurt us *twice*, by failing to stimulate additional supply, and by failing to moderate our demand. We'd get cheap gas, but less of it, and long lines for whatever we got.

In the wake of an economic dislocation like our current Debt-pression, many people want desperately to believe that government can solve the problem and keep it from happening again. It never works out that way, and by now we ought to know why. Making the right economic decision in any particular situation—that is, the decision that satisfies human need as abundantly as possible at the lowest cost—requires detailed knowledge of all the relevant considerations, and *that knowledge cannot be centralized. No one knows* how many loans banks should make or how many homes people should buy. It's not just that such knowledge doesn't exist in Washington; it's that such knowledge doesn't exist *anywhere*. We ought to stick with what works: liberty.

How Liberty Promotes Security

In my campaign literature, and on the cover of this book, I have reduced my platform to eight words: Less Government, More Liberty, More Prosperity, and More Security. Everyone seems to understand why "Less Government" means "More Liberty," and most people understand why "More Liberty" creates "More Prosperity." But some people wonder about the "More Security" part, particularly after a decade in which the federal government has repeatedly told us we have to surrender important civil liberties to stay safe. How exactly do less government and more liberty lead to more security? Let me mention just four ways.

First, economic liberty is what drives the creation of wealth, and it is the creation of wealth that allows people to live together peacefully. If you doubt that, and tend rather to think of money as the root of all evil, just imagine a society in which the amount of wealth were fixed. We cannot abolish scarcity by passing laws, so resources would still be scarce; that is, people would still want more than they have at any given time: more food, more shelter, more clothing, more services. But with the amount of wealth fixed, one could only obtain more by taking it from someone else. If no one could profit except at his neighbor's expense, we really would have a Hobbesian war of each against all.

The libertarian society, by contrast, is one in which people can cooperate to attain mutually beneficial aims. Voluntary trade makes both parties to the trade better off and generates greater material abundance. It is a win-win world. And this is true not only between citizens of the same country, but between countries as well. Liberty facilitates trade, trade promotes peace, and peace is the essential prerequisite for our security.

Enemies can be domestic as well as foreign, and liberty also provides us the greatest security against domestic enemies, people who would subvert our Constitution and arrogate power to themselves illegitimately. Our civil liberties prevent the peaceful accumulation of power that can be turned despotic. This is true most obviously of the liberties in the Bill of Rights, such as the Second and Tenth Amendments (which are typically supported by Republicans but not Democrats), the Fourth, Sixth, and Eighth Amendments (which are typically supported by Democrats but not Republicans), and the First Amendment (which is typically supported by everyone when the speaker or the religion is popular but tends to receive a much narrower reading when the speaker or the religion is unpopular). These liberties—*if we stick up for them vigorously enough*—prevent the national government from legislating "thought crimes," arresting people without charges, torturing confessions out of the innocent, or usurping the powers that were supposed to be exercised closer to home.

Unfortunately, Republicans didn't stick up for our civil liberties vigorously enough during the Bush years, and Democrats who were more vocal in 2006 seem to have lost either their voices or their integrity now that President Obama is the chief violator of our rights. Our security is now threatened not just by foreign nations or lawless thugs but by the internal threats posed by recent innovations like easier mechanisms for declaring martial law. Did you miss that one back in 2006? Do you think there's something wrong with a political culture in which such a law can be passed quietly? Even more recently, President Obama has ordered the summary assassination of a U.S. citizen, without formal charges or a trial, on mere suspicion of involvement with terrorist organizations. Can you think of any ways that might be misused by some future president? Like other wretched excesses of the "War on Terror," these entirely legal incursions on our liberties are part of a disturbing trend toward keeping the government safe by limiting the people instead of the other way around. We need a good dose of liberty to restore some security to the people.

Third, liberty promotes self-reliance and discourages the kind of dependency that can too easily be exploited for political control. My wife's Irish ancestors back in County Clare were thrown off their land in the nineteenth century because they refused to support the politician supported by their landlord. Standing up to that kind of pressure must have been hard, and it's not surprising that the story is remembered in the family more than 150 years later.

But one needn't have a long memory (or an Irish knack for grudge-holding) to understand this principle—because it happens today at all levels of our federal system. Federal money has long been used to coerce states into adopting policies dreamed up in Washington, no matter how ill-suited those policies are to the state's actual circumstances. (Remember when the speed limit in western deserts was 55 mph, just like the Washington-Baltimore corridor?) I have represented private educational institutions that were similarly coerced by the prospect of losing federal grant money. And more recently, coercive federal health care regulations have placed Catholic schools and hospitals in the uncomfortable position of having to choose between their deeply and sincerely held religious beliefs and the ability to continue serving the poor through their charitable institutions. The general rule is clear: When people pay to support the government, the people are in charge; when government pays to support the people, the politicians hold too many trump cards.

Fourth, liberty promotes sound foreign policy. I've written elsewhere about the virtues of a non-interventionist foreign policy, but let me add here that we are much more likely to catch ourselves overreaching abroad if we are still sensitive to government overreaching at home. When the war drums were beating for the invasion of Iraq, I noted the connection between free market principles and sound foreign policy. I tried in vain to help conservatives to see that if the government is not smart enough to know who ought to run General Motors (as we all agreed back then), it was probably not smart enough to know who should run Iraq. Little did I know that a few years later both Iraq *and* General Motors would have leadership changes dictated entirely by the President of the United States. I think that was no mere coincidence. Statist economic policies and imperialist foreign policies both presuppose that government planning is superior to individual liberty. That presupposition is poison, and we must purge ourselves of it.

Congress Fiddles While the Economy Burns

In late July 2010, with the Democratic Party firmly in control of the White House and both houses of Congress, the White House availed itself of the cynical and rather sophomoric tactic of releasing important but unflattering information on a Friday afternoon so that fewer people would notice it. What was the bad news? That budget deficits for Fiscal Years 2010 and 2011 were likely to be even higher than the $1.4 *trillion* we had to borrow to keep the lights on in Fiscal 2009.

[I fear that our use of the word "trillion" is beginning to hide the magnitude of our budget problems. For readers who aren't very good at math, $1.4 trillion is more properly written $1,400,000,000,000. It has 11 zeros. If you had that many dollar bills in a stack, it would reach almost halfway to the moon. If instead you made a carpet out of them, it would be about three times the size of Delaware.]

That day—July 23, 2010—has not been marked by historians, as far as I am aware, but I think it was quite significant. What mattered most, however, was not what happened that day; it was what happened next: Nothing.

I would like to tell you that Americans rose up in indignation, fired everyone in the House of Representatives (the body that appropriates money, you recall), and started over with a fresh group of representatives who understood the severity of our fiscal problems. I would like to tell you that in October 2010, when two little-known Libertarian candidates for the House unveiled a budget that actually achieved balance in just one year, and produced surpluses for all later years, a groundswell of support swept dozens of Libertarians into Congress. I would like to tell you that the Libertarians' stiff-spined leadership interrupted "business as usual" on Capitol Hill and put the country back on the road to a more peaceful and more prosperous tomorrow.

Unfortunately, that's not what happened.

Voters did deal a stinging rebuke to the Democratic Party, but the beneficiaries were the Republicans, who had received their own stinging rebukes in the two preceding elections. Some pundits expressed confidence that the Republicans had "learned their lesson" and that they would stick to their principles this time instead of falling back into their free-spending ways.

Unfortunately, that's not what happened either.

Instead, we know that Republicans came to town, talked tough, and approved spending *increases* together with tax cuts. A special bipartisan commission made some decent recommendations, but these were ignored immediately by both sides. The President's 2012 budget proposal failed to bring the budget into balance at any point in the next ten years. The Republicans' counterproposal, though less expensive than the President's, also permitted spending to rise and also failed to bring the budget into balance at any point in the next ten years. When our burgeoning national debt bumped up against the very generous limits our foreign creditors keep authorizing, Republicans and

Democrats joined hands and cast the hard votes necessary to . . . create another bipartisan committee. That committee also achieved nothing, to the surprise of no one.

And as I write this in the spring of 2012, it's all happening again. The President has once again submitted a budget that makes no serious effort to bring spending into line with revenues. He appears to regard deficits in the neighborhood of $1.3 trillion (that's $1,300,000,000,000) as "the new normal." Republican budgetmeister Paul Ryan has countered with a budget that costs about $5 trillion less over the next *ten years,* but which would not manage to balance our budget until approximately 2040.

It's hard to write anything about this because it's hard to believe it's necessary. Isn't it obvious that we simply can't continue this way? Wasn't it already obvious when the deficits were less than half as large as they are now? All that has happened in the interim is that the change we so obviously need has become harder, and we have less time to effect it.

But since the point has so far been lost on my own senators and congressman, and on most others, let me offer four brief observations on budget policy and budget politics.

First, note how large these deficits are *in percentage terms.* It's not just that we're borrowing over $1,300,000,000,000 per year; it's that we're borrowing more than *40 cents out of every dollar we spend.* For every three dollars the federal government takes in, Congress has spent not just an extra nickel or even an extra quarter, but an extra *two bucks.* In other words, they're not even close, and they haven't been for years!

Why does this matter? Partly because it tells us that no one's really trying very hard to balance the budget; it is as if no one really remembers that ideally the expenditures should be lower than the revenues. No one in Congress seems to remember what zero means anymore. (It means, "Stop spending.") Obviously, the correct response to this on our part is to fire Congress.

But perhaps more importantly, it also tells us that it's ludicrous for people to approach our budget problems by talking about how to save money here and there on existing programs. The only way to limit the size and cost of government is to limit the number of things we ask government to do. The only way to cut our government back down to a size we can live with is to eliminate all the extraneous programs that our founders never intended for a national government to do in the first place. The road to fiscal responsibility in 2013 and beyond runs right through Article I of our Constitution.

My second brief observation is that it's no mere coincidence that these gargantuan deficits became routine during a period in which Congress suddenly decided that the job of passing a budget each year was optional. If your budget were this out of whack—and if you or your spouse is out of work, it may be— then surely the first thing you would do is sit down and *make a plan*. Somehow expenditures need to be brought into balance with revenues, and there's no budget fairy that will do that for us while we're sleeping (or passing expensive entitlements, or even trashing the first amendment by passing new regulations of campaign speech). Saving money—*big money—did I mention that we're talking about $1,300,000,000,000 per year?*—takes thought; it takes effort. Without a blueprint for saving money, is it any wonder that no money was saved?

Remember this in November: In the face of a looming fiscal disaster capable of shaking the very foundations of our national government, our current representatives—Republicans and Democrats alike—have done *nothing. They didn't even take a shot at it*. Again, obviously, the correct response to this on our part is to fire Congress.

Third, there is a lot of talk in Washington about "reducing the deficit," or putting the budget on a "glide path" that supposedly will result in a balanced budget sometime in the distant future. President Obama's former budget chief once bragged that he was on track to cut the budget deficit in half before the end of President Obama's first term. As the President would say, "Let me be clear": Cutting the deficit in half is an idiotic goal. We have got to stop thinking of budget deficits as if they have no more long-term significance than last night's baseball score. Every year in which *any* deficit exists raises the national debt, and it's the national debt that determines how much of next year's budget gets soaked up in interest payments we can't do anything about. Even in the unlikely event that deficit spending in 2013 can be held as low as the $900,000,000,000 the President projects, *that will be really, really bad.* This is not a good-news-bad-news story. There is no silver lining.

Finally, the persistent use—by Democrats and Republicans—of gimmicks like ten-year budget forecasts and bipartisan commissions is nothing short of contemptible. The ten-year budget plans are a fraud on the public, because no one lives in years two through ten; we live in year one, year after year. And as for bipartisan committees, we already have one that's supposed to balance the budget every year. It's called Congress, and we pay an awful lot to keep it in session. If the people we've been sending to Congress for years and years, Democrats and Republicans alike, are collectively too timid, too lazy, or too incompetent to even try to tackle the single biggest problem we face as a nation, then it's high time for us to send different people to Congress.

People sometimes debate hypothetical questions about how far we would go to make a terrorist tell us the location of a ticking time bomb. But for Pete's sake, there's a debt bomb ticking loudly right inside the Capitol at this very moment, and no one in the Congressional leadership seems to care! How much time do they think we have?

This is not complicated. We need to spend less. Much less. Starting right now.

Exercisers, Dieters, and Real Fiscal Fitness: A Field Guide to Budget Politics

If there is any silver lining in the fiscal storm clouds that threaten our economic future, it is this: Virtually every candidate for federal office this November will be talking about the importance of reducing federal budget deficits. But ironically, the proposals most likely to lead us back to fiscal responsibility will be the ones that are primarily motivated by something else: the desire to get government off our backs.

Broadly speaking, we can expect "deficit reduction" proposals to fall into three main camps. In one camp we have the Exercisers. The Exercisers believe in *very* active government, so they are very reluctant to do anything even to slow the growth of existing programs, and any actual reduction in government spending is out of the question as far as they are concerned. Consequently, the Exercisers' most visible proposals will be to increase taxes, at least on the "rich." They may also propose some spending restraint, like freezing discretionary spending and "paying for" any new spending with offsetting program cuts or tax hikes, but these proposals will be mostly for show; the fine print will always render these ornamental bits of "restraint" mathematically immaterial.

As a result, the Exercisers don't really propose to balance the budget themselves; they want to wait around for *us* to do it, by working harder and producing more income to tax. We are the real deficit reducers in this scenario; we change the deficit equation by working hard enough to boost federal tax receipts. In fact, many Exercisers think that boosting tax revenue is so important that it justifies spending *more* money now, on the theory that a bigger government spending more of our money will actually "stimulate" the private economy and create more jobs.

Most of those who oppose the Exercisers will be Dieters. The Dieters treat excessive federal spending the way many of us treat excessive eating: as something we need to moderate but which it's not practical to reduce very much. The Dieters will trim here and there, and they'll be conspicuous in their refusal to pass new spending programs. Unfortunately for the Dieters, we need to cut spending by more than 40 percent to get it down to the level of tax receipts, and the Dieters can't bring themselves to propose that.

Say this for the Dieters, though: They know we need to reduce government spending rather than just sending more Ho-Ho's to Washington. This will lead the Dieters to oppose any measure that raises new tax revenue from any source. But without deep reductions in federal spending, the Dieters are playing almost as much of a waiting game as the Exercisers. Again, with the Dieters in power, the only real hope for a balanced budget will be for *us* to balance it, by working harder and producing a larger total output from which government can take its cut. Dieters don't publicly endorse the Exercisers' belief that government can stimulate the private sector by spending more, but they tend to find plenty of other reasons for government to spend more, particularly on the military and particularly for big spending projects in their own home districts.

The third group, by far the smallest right now, is the group I have sometimes called the Zeros. The Zeros know that we're not supposed to have a budget deficit at all; that when the Treasury gets to zero, Congress is supposed to stop spending. The Zeros also know that zero happens to be the correct amount that should be appropriated for many federal programs. And when they find such a program, Zeros enthusiastically propose to zero it out. You might know the Zeros better by their more common name: Libertarians.

Libertarians propose deep cuts in federal spending, driven by the complete elimination of programs that are deemed unnecessary, unhelpful, unconstitutional, or just too expensive. Libertarians would never dream of submitting a ten-year budget showing ten straight deficits, as the other two groups do. If elected in sufficient numbers, Libertarians would balance the budget in the very next fiscal year.

Why do the Libertarians show so much more fiscal discipline than the other two groups? Largely for reasons that have nothing to do with budget math. Unlike the other two groups, Libertarians do not accept the basic premise that government spending is good for us. Libertarians don't think of federal spending as a necessity for our economic health (like the Exercisers) or as a sweet-tasting treat (like the Dieters). We Libertarians think very little federal spending makes voters better off, and quite a bit of it makes us worse off—not (merely) because we can't afford it but because it interferes with our personal and economic liberty. Libertarians find it intolerable that Congress dictates how we work, play, save, invest, hire and fire, and even eat. We're tougher on government spending because we think most government spending would be bad for us even if there were no budget deficit.

Libertarians are for reducing taxes as well, because a smaller government requires less revenue. But many Libertarians are also happy to eliminate special-interest tax credits that have been stuffed into the revenue side of the budget. Unlike Dieters, we object to government coercion in the form of tax credits just as much as we object to government coercion in the form of costly regulatory programs. Given the opportunity to replace the income tax with some other tax that Congress couldn't use to manipulate the economy, many Libertarians would jump at the chance.

Thus, while almost every candidate will claim to be in favor of fiscal discipline this November, it really matters *what kind* of discipline they favor. Both Exercisers and Dieters share the assumption that government spending is presumptively good, while the taxation necessary to pay for those programs is presumptively bad. No one should be surprised that the clash of these views produces a result that *sounds* a lot like gridlock, but is actually the ideal bipartisan compromise: more spending, without paying for anywhere near all of it.

The path toward real, long-term fiscal fitness lies instead with the Libertarians. Voters who genuinely want fiscal discipline may get it only if they focus first on liberating our economy from decades of federal micromanagement.

Enough Blame to Go Around

Most of the people in my family are Republicans, and sometimes they chide me for being too hard on Republicans in general and President Bush in particular. One of them points out that budget deficits were declining in Fiscal Years 2005, 2006, and 2007, before Democrats took over control of Congress. (The Democratic Congress elected in November 2006 took office approximately three months into Fiscal Year 2007.) Since Fiscal 2007, however, deficits have soared to the levels that make financial collapse a real possibility today. So is it really fair for me to blame Republicans and Democrats alike? Haven't the Democrats been worse?

There is no question that deficits got worse when Democrats took control of Congress. Nonetheless, I believe Republicans deserve every bit of criticism I give them and more, based on their fiscal performance during the Bush administration. Here are five reasons why.

First, the Bush administration began with an annual budget surplus and quickly squandered it. This destroyed any chance of drawing some fiscal discipline from the idea that we did not want to return to the bad old days of deficit spending. After years of deficit spending, we had a few years in which it was actually possible to re-learn the meaning of zero in budget discussions, and promote a strong political consensus that we need always to keep our annual deficit numbers in the black. It was the chance of a generation if not a lifetime, and the Republicans blew it. The fact that they did this with full awareness of the demographic time bomb that has been widely discussed since my own adolescence puts the Republicans' misrule in a particularly unflattering light.

Second, the deficits during President Bush's term were caused by an enormous spending spree that was entirely within the ruling party's control. Apologists for President Bush and his fellow Republicans like to point to the role of the unexpected, starting with the attacks of September 11, 2001 and the ensuing recession—and it's true that federal revenues went down instead of up in FY 2002 and 2003. But that excuse overlooks the fact that President Bush's very first budget proposed significant and sustained spending increases as far as the eye could see—and that budget was submitted to Congress in February 2001, before 9/11 or any recession. Nor was this simply a case of bad leadership from the White House; actual federal spending approved by the Republican Congress was even higher than President Bush proposed. In fact, if we look at actual federal spending from 2001 to 2009, the trajectory is not significantly different from the trajectory projected by President Obama for the next five years.

Third, once we look at spending and deficits together, we see that the declining deficits of 2005-2007 were caused not by any sort of fiscal restraint by Republicans, but rather by growing federal tax revenues in an economy the Federal Reserve was obligingly inflating into the bubble that burst in 2008. Spending growth was more or less constant. This helps to show why the focus in deficit reduction has always got to be on the spending side. Economies go through good times and bad; revenues go up and they go down. We need to run surpluses and pay down debt in the good times instead of pretending the debt isn't there. Given the size of our current debt, that's unlikely to change for decades, if ever.

Fourth, as I have argued in an earlier essay on deficits, no one ever deserves credit for making deficits smaller, because any deficit means by definition that we are moving in the wrong direction, becoming more indebted. I have said that we need to stop thinking of annual deficit numbers the way we think of the score of last night's ballgame. What I mean is that when a team loses a ballgame, it's completely over and the important thing is to forget about it and do better next time. The poor showing in a single game is not without consequences— it's harder to win a league title after a loss than it would have been with a win—but Tuesday's game does not ordinarily affect Wednesday's. That's not true with deficits, because of the national debt. The 2006 deficit cost us extra money in 2007, and we have been raising our own borrowing costs more and more in every single year since then—digging ourselves a deeper and deeper hole.

Fifth, the annual deficit figures from 2001-2009 do not capture the full measure of the Republicans' fiscal recklessness, because some of the policy choices made during those years effectively committed us to spending more money in the future. In other words, foreign wars and expensive domestic programs are two more things that are not like last night's ballgame. As long as government spending grows—as it always does under Republicans and Democrats alike—every Congress finds austerity harder than the Congress that preceded it, because it's always harder to cut existing programs than to vote against creating new ones. That doesn't excuse Democrats for the budget-busting they've done since 2007. But it does prevent Republicans from pretending that the choices they made years ago aren't part of the problem we still face today. Many government policies are just too foolish to permit us to judge them one year at a time.

Some Republicans might object that by 2012 the performance of Republicans during the Bush administration has become ancient history, and that today's Republicans are much more fiscally responsible. But where is the evidence for this assertion? After the Republican Party recaptured control of the House in 2010, the cable channels were full of speculation about the big changes coming to Washington. I predicted spending would actually increase, and of course it did (though you'd be hard pressed to find much news of that on the cable channels). So even voters who were inclined in 2010 to credit Republican claims that they had repented of their free-spending ways must finally confront the truth: Republicans like big government too; they differ from Democrats regarding shape, not size.

Some readers may wonder whether this question of blame really matters. I think it does, particularly in light of the huge rejections of Republican rule that took place in 2006 and 2008 and the huge rejection of Democratic rule that took place in 2010. We must be extremely clear about what we are rejecting when we "throw the bums out." We certainly need to throw out incumbents who have voted to give away hundreds of billions of dollars without seeming to notice that we're broke. But we can't simply allow the two major parties to take turns screwing things up. We need to replace free-spending incumbents with genuine fiscal conservatives who really want to shrink the federal government. As long as the Republican party is under the leadership of people who were all complicit in the Bush administration's lousy fiscal performance, I think voters need to look elsewhere for the right person.

Is the Libertarian Party Really Different?

In an earlier essay, we tried to place Libertarians somewhere on the popular but not-very-informative left-right "political spectrum." As part of that effort, we saw how Libertarians differ from Democrats and Republicans. But the many voters who have learned to hate both major parties often wonder: How can *any* party be trusted? Why should anyone believe the Libertarian Party is different?

I love this question, because it was my question for many years. The short answer is that while most parties exist to promote the electoral success of their candidates, the Libertarian Party exists to promote liberty, win or lose. We would rather be principled than powerful. And that's what makes it safe to trust us with power.

As we have seen, the Libertarian combination of views looks like an ungainly hybrid to people who are used to arranging political views along a single left-to-right axis. By combining fiscally conservative and apparently "pro-business" views on economic matters with socially tolerant and anti-war views,

Libertarians can look to some people as if they are trying to sew an elephant's head onto a donkey's torso.

But if we pay closer attention, we see that the part of each major party that Libertarians combine is the *principled* part. Libertarians oppose government interference with individual liberty for any purpose other than to protect the person or property of another individual. This is known as the "non-aggression principle," and it is more fundamental for Libertarians than any particular plank of the party's platform. Thus, what may look at first blush like a mixing and matching of standard R and D positions is actually a much more consistent application of a principled preference for individual liberty over government coercion.

Neither major party accepts the non-aggression principle, but that's not the only way they differ from the Libertarian Party. In practice, there is *no* political principle to which *either* major party is committed more strongly than it is committed to winning elections. The two major political parties exist, first and foremost, to win elections. They are private clubs that exist for the purpose of electing their members, and if they believe that changing their policy positions, their political philosophies, or their demographic composition will help them elect more members of their club, they will make those changes in a heartbeat. This has actually happened many times in the history of the Republicans and the Democrats, as any good history of those parties makes clear. (For anyone who wants to check this out, I can recommend Lewis Gould's *Grand Old Party*.)

Libertarians are different. If you don't believe this, go to the Libertarian Party's website, www.lp.org, and try to join the party. Before the party accepts your membership (or your money), you will be asked to take the following pledge: "I certify that I oppose the initiation of force to achieve political or social goals." Libertarians don't all agree on exactly what

90

the pledge means, and there is sometimes room for reasonable minds to differ about what counts as protection of person or property rather than a "political or social goal." The value of the pledge, though, is that it anchors the debate around a principle that is much more protective of individual liberty than the perpetual, poll-driven pursuit of power practiced by the major parties.

The first time I thought about joining the Libertarian Party, I stopped at the non-aggression pledge. It was so broad that, even if it sounded good in theory, I wasn't sure it would succeed in practice. After a few more years of watching the clown show we call Congress, I came to understand that it's the unchecked pursuit of electoral power that is the ultimate practical failure. After spending years as an "unaffiliated" voter (that's what we call "independents" here in Maryland), it now seems to me that the pledge is the only reason I could consider joining any party again. It is the pledge, and the party's principled commitment to non-aggression, that makes the Libertarian Party more trustworthy than the others.

Libertarianism and the Environment

I'm an environmentalist. I spend several weeks each summer in New York's Adirondack State Park, enjoying the mountains, lakes, and rivers in that beautiful place. But I'm against "cap and trade" proposals and most other ideas for new federal environmental laws and regulations, because they don't work. Environmental protection has been dominated for decades by large government regulatory initiatives, but experience shows that government regulation can't *and doesn't* protect the environment as effectively as private ownership and a strong dose of civil liability for actual environmental damage.

In the short term, I favor waiving the government's sovereign immunity in environmental litigation, so that government is fully accountable for the environmental harms it covers. In the longer term, I favor a transition away from government regulation, which doesn't work, and toward strict enforcement of property rights so that people can sue for restitution from polluters who put things in our air, water, and soil that we don't want there.

The first thing to understand about environmental protection is that government is the main culprit. Our federal government (particularly the military) is the nation's largest polluter, and a great deal of pollution by commercial enterprises occurs on government lands that are being poorly managed. Why are government lands poorly managed? Because government managers do not take care of them as well as a private owner would. The Izaak Walton League, the Nature Conservancy, the Sierra Club—any of these would manage our national parks better than the federal government does.

If you doubt this, consider Louisiana's Rainey Preserve, a bird sanctuary owned by the National Audubon Society. Despite the environmental sensitivity, Audubon allowed oil and gas drilling in the Rainey Preserve from the 1940s to the 1990s. Why? Because Audubon *as a private owner* was able to weigh the risks and rewards for itself and was able to include important environmental protections in its contracts with the oil and gas companies. For example, Audubon forbade the companies from drilling during nesting season. That cost Audubon some revenue, but presumably Audubon was happy to forgo the extra money in return for protecting the snowy egret. And Audubon's ability to custom-tailor the drilling rights in this way, and monitor compliance with the conditions in the contract, allowed Audubon to earn $25 million from oil and gas drilling that could then be used for Audubon's many other conservation programs.

By contrast, when the question of drilling in the Arctic National Wildlife Refuge arose in the mid-1990s, Audubon was in vehement opposition. Some may suspect hypocrisy, but to a libertarian it makes perfect sense. Audubon had good reason to fear that federal management of drilling in the ANWR would not be as environmentally sensitive as Audubon's. Furthermore, as a non-owner, Audubon could have no assurance that the revenue from drilling in the ANWR would go toward conservation (or any other worthwhile cause for that matter). With no environmental upside and a significant risk of harm from government mismanagement, opposition to ANWR drilling was probably an easy call for Audubon. (For this example I am indebted to Richard L. Stroup and his book, *Eco-Nomics: What Everyone Should Know About Economics and the Environment*.)

Audubon's opposition to the ANWR drilling was vindicated by the 2010 offshore drilling tragedy in the Gulf of Mexico, which had Big Government's fingerprints all over it. First, Congress capped Big Oil's liability for spills, so that Big Oil wouldn't have to pay as much for liability insurance. But that meant that Big Oil also didn't have as much economic incentive to be careful with the Gulf ecosystem, nor was there an insurance carrier on board deepwater rigs to make sure that best practices were being followed. Next, a federal agency that had been completely "captured" by the industry it was supposed to regulate paid far less attention to safety than Audubon would have—less even than a private insurer would have, if BP had insured against environmental harm instead of getting Congress to cap its liability. We all know how the story ended. From a libertarian perspective, we should never have expected any other ending once the government got involved.

In addition, private ownership protects the little guy far better than bureaucratic rulemaking can. If you don't like the stuff an upwind polluter is dropping on your property, you should be able to sue for the damage it causes, and the fact that you don't want it on your property should be reason enough for the polluter to keep it off. If the polluter wants the right to drop stuff there, he should have to pay you for that. You, of course, should have every right to refuse. But with government regulation, a supposedly "expert" agency starts a rulemaking and takes testimony from scientists (paid for by the polluters) about whether the unwanted pollutant is harmful, and if so whether it is really harmful or just a little bit harmful. Quite apart from the fact that you can't afford as many scientists as the polluters can, what gets lost in all the bureaucracy is that *it's your land and you don't want pollution on it*. In a libertarian society, that should be enough.

The big-government approach to environmental issues hurts us in other ways as well. President Obama's decision to delay the Keystone oil pipeline from Canada on environmental grounds is already costing us jobs and diminishing our access to oil from our most stable and most geopolitically compatible neighbor. Similarly, the policy of steering government money toward the so-called "green energy" sector has been marred by commercial failures and significant losses for taxpayers—and it has distorted the incentives for the green energy companies themselves, as such government largesse always does.

Libertarianism and Non-Discrimination Laws

In 2010, Kentucky Senate candidate (now Senator) Rand Paul drew unfavorable press attention for his remarks about the Civil Rights Act of 1964. Even though Paul is a Republican, his libertarian sympathies led some people who had never paid much attention to libertarians to ask whether we are soft on racial bigotry. Do libertarians really believe that all civil rights legislation was wrong? Would we repeal the laws protecting voting rights and desegregating public accommodations if we could?

For "the short answer," let me start with Section 3.5 of the Libertarian Party platform, which "condemn[s] bigotry as irrational and repugnant" and adds, "Government should not deny or abridge any individual's rights based on sex, wealth, race, color, creed, age, national origin, personal habits, political preference or sexual orientation." The preamble likewise states "that respect for individual rights is the essential precondition for a free and prosperous world." Libertarians want a government that is *radically neutral* toward its citizens. Libertarians therefore proudly support laws like the Voting Rights Act that protect political equality, as well as those provisions of the

Civil Rights Act that banned discrimination in voter registration practices and prohibited racial segregation in government agencies, public schools, and other public facilities.

But what about the part of the Civil Rights Act that banned *private* discrimination? That's where Libertarians draw attention to the downsides of government intervention. Laws banning private discrimination can be justified on libertarian principles, but probably only as a response to the historically unique issue of race. To understand the pros and cons of anti-discrimination laws, let's look a little more closely at our Constitution and our history than either Senator Paul or his critics did.

Race in our history

The actual history of the fight for civil rights in this country is not the good-government fairy tale in which some cable celebrities seem to believe. Their story seems to be that 1964 was the year an enlightened government finally ended 350 years of private discrimination by immoral individuals. That is wildly misleading; in fact, it's just wrong. The truth is that during those 350 years *black Americans were victimized first and foremost by governments*. *Governments* treated African-American slaves as sub-human until 1865. *Governments* treated runaway slaves like lost property that had to be returned. Nearly a century after the Civil War, *governments* still treated black Americans like second-class citizens, and *governments* looked the other way and refused to protect black Americans from violent attacks on their lives, liberty, and property.

Meanwhile, classical liberals like William Lloyd Garrison— people who today would be called libertarians—agitated privately for racial justice. These proto-libertarians attacked slavery as "man-stealing," a violation of the slave's self-ownership. And the latter-day civil rights movement behind Martin Luther King was a model of powerful non-violent witness by individual citizens who refused to accept the injustice of their laws. Governments did not lead that movement; governments were more often aiming the fire hoses and loosing the dogs.

The story of the Civil Rights Act, then, is not that pure-hearted legislators finally prevailed over wicked owners of segregated lunch counters. It is that individuals with a thirst for equal justice under the law put their very lives on the line for racial equality, and in so doing they finally shamed Congress into exercising its constitutional power to stop *state governments* from treating blacks as second-class citizens.

Race in our Constitution

Sadly, most non-lawyers have never heard of Congress's express constitutional power to secure political equality for Americans of all races, but that power was granted to Congress at the end of the Civil War, in the Fourteenth Amendment. Section 1 of that Amendment finally extended citizenship to black Americans and prohibited states from depriving freed slaves of the full equality to which they were entitled. Section 5 of that Amendment stated, with remarkable breadth, "The Congress shall have power to enforce, by appropriate legislation, the provisions of this article." *That's* what the Civil Rights Act of 1964 was doing.

Unfortunately, Congress also claimed, unnecessarily, that the Act could be justified as a regulation of interstate commerce—and that's what has raised concerns among people who favor small government. Constitutional law typically respects precedent, so each expansive interpretation of government power in one case paves the way for further expansions in other cases. An expansive use of the power to remedy racial discrimination can easily be limited to the historically unique issue of race; but an expansive use of the commerce power necessarily expands

Congressional power over activities that have nothing to do with race or any kind of discrimination.

For example, if Congressional power over commerce is broad enough to justify laws that force sellers to sell to certain buyers, then it is presumably also broad enough to force buyers to buy from certain sellers. And there's nothing hypothetical about that; in the spring of 2010, we saw Congress invoke its commerce power to require all Americans to buy compulsory health insurance. Likewise, if Congress can regulate the racial composition of a business's employees under its commerce power, then Congress can presumably also use the commerce power to regulate what those employees are allowed to earn—another encroachment on economic liberty that is unfortunately no longer hypothetical. Other bills in recent years have relied on the commerce power in order to place federal limits on how much carbon we can emit, or how fast we can drive. Thus, Congress's invocation of its commerce power to pass the Civil Rights Act was pregnant with the possibility of even more intrusion on private action in the years ahead. That would not have been true if Congress had relied only on its power to implement the Fourteenth Amendment.

The price of purging prejudice

With that historical and constitutional context, we can finally get to the heart of the controversy over Rand Paul's remarks. No true libertarian can be soft on racial bigotry; we are zealous in our defense of each individual's right to equal justice under law. But we pay dearly with our liberty if we cede to Congress the power to compel economic transactions between unwilling participants. Many libertarians believe that the Civil Rights Act's prohibition on government-sponsored segregation would have been sufficient to end private discrimination throughout the south. We can't know for sure, but if so then it was unwise to expand federal power that way—unwise because it was unnecessary. And in any event, it was unwise to expand the federal *commerce* power when a more specific power to combat racial discrimination was already in the Constitution. Our historical experience of how power corrupts tells us that the individual liberties of all Americans would be safer today if we all recognized that the Civil Rights Act was *entirely about racial equality*, and was in no way typical of the kind of power Congress should exercise over private businesses.

Racial discrimination is our nation's original sin; the greatest stain on our founding and the cause of our bloodiest war. We are a better society because of civil rights legislation—not as good a society as if racial discrimination had never existed, but that option was not on the menu for anyone alive today. The libertarian insight is that our willingness to let government depart from strict neutrality—to let government be nonneutral toward bigots—set a precedent that made government more powerful and our liberty less secure. Acknowledging that, and showing an appropriate wariness about government power, is the least we owe the memory of those who suffered so long under government-sponsored racial aggression.

Pro-Life and Pro-Liberty

Many people express surprise when they learn that I have pro-life views on the legality of abortion. How, they wonder, can a Libertarian be in favor of having such a personal issue decided by the government? I'm happy to address this, because I think the answer tells us a lot about libertarianism, as well as about abortion as a moral and political issue.

Recall that Libertarians believe the central purpose of government is to protect the person and property of every member of the community from violence initiated by others. Similarly, we believe that the central limitation on government is that it should *not* initiate force against any person *except* to protect the person or property of another member of the community.

For Libertarians, then, as for most people, the very first question we need to resolve is: How many persons does abortion involve? If abortion is simply a surgical procedure performed on a pregnant woman—one person—then libertarian principles require that the woman be free to do as she pleases without government interference. But if abortion is the deliberate killing of one person for the benefit of another, then it lies at the very heart of all that governments are instituted to prevent and abortion should be legal only when the mother's life or health is itself in danger.

Some people frame the question as "whether life begins at conception. I don't find that very helpful. "Life" began billions of years ago. What matters is when a particular *person* came into being; a singular, uniquely precious, human life distinct from any other. Obviously a fetus must be alive or else there could be no question of killing it. Just as obviously the life is human; with distinctively human chromosomes, we know it is not a puppy. And finally, the human life in the mother's womb is genetically distinct from the mother; it is *not* simply a part of the mother's body, or it would have the same DNA fingerprint.

A majority of Libertarians reject this argument, but the party's official platform plank on abortion (section 1.4) takes as neutral a pro-choice view as it is possible to take: "Recognizing that abortion is a sensitive issue and that people can hold good-faith views on all sides, we believe that government should be kept out of the matter, leaving the question to each person for their conscientious consideration." This is not very protective of unborn children, but at least our party does not trumpet the right to an abortion as a fundamental civil liberty.

This is not the first time in American history that a political controversy has boiled down to the question of who counts as a person. Howard Fineman, in his thoughtful survey of *The Thirteen American Arguments,* reckons "Who is a person?" to be Argument Number One. It is the argument we have whenever we are on the cusp of expanding liberty, whether to religious dissenters or to former slaves or to formerly subservient women.

In the antebellum south, racial subjugation was routinely defended by otherwise decent people who insisted that black and white people were different not just in color but in kind; that they belonged to different "races." In hindsight, we know that those otherwise decent people were deceived by appearances; genetic research now establishes that there is only one race and it's human.

Decades later the question was not slavery but segregation. Many of us have heard the ringing affirmation, "Our Constitution is color-blind, and neither knows nor tolerates classes among citizens." Some know that the sentence was penned in *dissent* from a Supreme Court decision upholding a Louisiana law that required racial segregation of railway cars. *Plessy v. Ferguson,* 163 U.S. 537, 559 (1896). What most people do not know is that just three paragraphs after he declared our Constitution color-blind, Justice Harlan went on to describe "the Chinese race" as "so different from our own that we do not permit those belonging to it to become citizens of the United States." 163 U.S. at 561. I wish I could ask Justice Harlan why he thought Chinese people "so different" that even a colorblind Constitution afforded them no protection. But all I can do is recognize that even a judge who saw the injustice of government-mandated segregation with brilliant clarity, a full 50 years before the rest of the Supreme Court, was still fallible enough to botch the same moral question three paragraphs later.

I think of this when I hear an abortion-rights advocate describe a living, growing fetus as nothing more than a "bag of cells" or something like that. We're *all* bags of cells; the question is whether some bags of cells have less right to live than others. I think all of us, but perhaps especially Libertarians, should resist that conclusion.

I recognize, of course, that many good people disagree with my analysis of the abortion question, just as many good people disagreed with Justice Harlan. I can try to persuade, but I cannot force them to change their minds. And I know that in the end the law will follow whatever social consensus we are able to develop.

That's what happened with racial segregation. *Plessy v. Ferguson* was not so misguided as to freeze the legality of racial segregation into place once and for all. States were free to repeal their segregation laws. Private citizens were free to integrate their workplaces, their neighborhoods, and their personal relationships. The culture could correct itself, and it did.

By contrast, the Court's landmark 1973 abortion decision in *Roe v. Wade* effectively torpedoed the democratic sorting and sifting that had been taking place throughout the 1960s, and left almost no room for legitimate debate on the fundamentals in the 40 years that have passed since the case was decided. Whichever way our society eventually resolves this question, it is very hard for me to see how we can move forward until *Roe v. Wade* is overturned and the legality of abortion is once again a matter of state law.

Do We Need Consumer Product Safety Regulation?

Government regulations are so pervasive that many people assume without question both that the regulations are helpful and that they are necessary. However, once we challenge these assumptions, we see that government regulation is frequently not only unnecessary, but futile or even counterproductive. Rather than pretending that government always knows what's good for us and what's not, Libertarians prefer to let individual consumers decide which products they trust. Not every product on the market is safe—but that's true even of products the government has declared to be safe, and we're better off knowing that the responsibility rests with us.

A recent question I received about expanding the FDA's role in regulating cosmetics illustrates the point. The question came with a link to a video called "The Story of Cosmetics," by filmmaker and activist Annie Leonard. The argument of the film is that there are too many toxins in personal care products like shampoos and deodorants, and that the FDA should be given new authority to ban the use of toxic ingredients in these products. The video is well done, and I really encourage people to consider the "toxins in, toxins out" message when they're buying cosmetics and other household products. But the video claims that additional FDA regulation will be more effective than relying on consumers to make good choices. That argument just doesn't wash.

First, "The Story of Cosmetics" assumes that FDA regulation will make our shampoos safer, even though we're talking about regulations that have yet to be written, sometime in the future. But the same video also argues that the problem with current regulations is that cosmetics makers have captured the government regulatory process and have subverted it so that toxic chemicals are allowed in. So why should we expect regulation to work better the second time? We shouldn't.

It doesn't even matter why the manufacturers escaped regulation the first time around. Maybe industry produced scientific evidence that genuinely convinced Congress or the FDA's experts that there was no need for regulation. Or maybe the case for regulation was pretty strong, but industry prevailed due to sheer political muscle. Either way, there is good reason to expect the same result the second time around.

Second, the video asserts that we cannot address this problem *without* FDA regulation. But here the video contradicts itself by pointing out that "green chemistry" for consumer products is already a flourishing field. Why is it flourishing? *Because there's a market for non-toxic consumer products!* Tom's of Maine, Seventh Generation, Kiss My Face—there are lots of brands on the market that attempt to make us clean and shiny without using toxic chemicals. What government agency should we thank for that? None. It was private enterprise.

The video suggests private enterprise won't work here because a single consumer can't affect what Procter & Gamble puts into

its shampoo. But when the video turns to the lawmaking process, suddenly the narrator is one of many people who all want
the same thing. Where were all these people when P&G was
figuring out what to put in the shampoo? Why wouldn't a
group of consumers big enough to get Congress's attention be
big enough to get P&G's? Shouldn't it be *easier* to get *P&G's*
attention, since P&G makes lots of shampoos without requiring
any one of them to be favored by more than 50% of all voters?

Of course government doesn't require the assent of 50% of all
voters either; it responds to small groups of people who are zealous enough and influential enough to pull the right legislative
and regulatory levers—the infamous "special interests." Thus,
if government does start regulating your deodorant, it will not
be because you and I and all our neighbors joined hands and
decided to rein in P&G. If government starts regulating your
deodorant, it will be because a relatively small group of people
who focus on the toxicity of consumer products think they can
choose your deodorant better than you can. Libertarians don't
think that's a good enough reason to regulate.

Third, we can never eliminate the risk of mistake, so individuals should have the freedom to balance risks as they see fit.
Governments may approve unsafe products, or ban safe products, or conduct decades of tests that fail to produce complete
consensus, as was the case with aspartame. Statists argue that
this uncertainty makes it necessary for government to take the
decision away from us because we have imperfect information.
But that ignores the existence of videos like the one I'm criti-
quing—which in fact does an *excellent* job of informing us about
potential risks. It's true that I can't evaluate toxicity on my
own, but it's not true that government is the only source I can
turn to for help.

Moreover, this problem of imperfect information is not limited to the decisions we make as consumers. If I'm not smart

enough to know which shampoo ingredients are toxic, then I'm *also* not smart enough to know whether an FDA action permitting these chemicals is a good decision or a bad one. That means I have to rely on others for my information either way; the only difference is that with the free market I end up with the ability to weigh the information, make my own decision, and live with the consequences. I may be left with an uncertain and somewhat dissatisfying tradeoff, with pros and cons for each choice, but that's a lousy excuse for asking the government to take the choice away from me.

Finally, some argue that leaving the market unregulated will mean that rich people can buy more expensive "green" products that not everyone can afford. But wait: If price is the only reason someone is currently not buying a green shaving cream, how is government regulation going to help? Government regulation will not make the green product cheaper; on the contrary, it will make the green product more expensive, both by adding new costs of doing business and by removing marketplace alternatives that the FDA doesn't like. Thus, the real effect of regulation here is to *make the average Joe spend more on green shaving cream whether he wants to or not.* Folks who want FDA regulations are saying the average Joe is a fool not to spend his money on green shaving cream now, so they're going to remove other shaving creams from the market to protect him from his own folly.

But what if the average Joe is not a fool? What if he just thinks other items in his budget (more food, more organic food, a nicer apartment, cholesterol medication) are more important? What if the right shaving cream for Joe to buy depends on what's important to Joe? Libertarians think we ought to let Joe sort that out.

Big Government and Big Business

We've seen how liberty creates prosperity, and how government interference with our economic liberty distorts investment decisions and makes us worse off. But some people think we need a strong government to protect us from powerful economic interests. That theory sounds reasonable—if you don't know what it's like to run a business and you don't pay any attention to how government works in practice.

But in practice, even large businesses don't have anything like the power screenwriters give them in the movies. As the late Harry Browne used to say, "No matter how big a business is, you don't have to deal with it; there's always an alternative—including not buying at all." Show me a business that treats its customers the way the Post Office and the Motor Vehicle Administration do, and I'll show you a stock you should short.

And in practice, career politicians and industry regulators almost always use government to advance the interests of the largest and most politically connected businesses rather than their smaller competitors or their customers. Indeed, when I ask people to give me an example of a business from which they need to be protected, most reach for *government-sponsored* monopolies, like the old AT&T. Occasionally someone mentions a firm that figured prominently in the credit meltdown of late 2008, but those firms would no longer exist if it weren't for their *political* clout. As a purely economic matter, the free market was all set to discipline those firms with bankruptcy until the government stepped in.

The truth is that government tends not to protect us from economically powerful businesses, but rather to protect politically powerful businesses from us. Licensing laws are a great example. If you live in a city, you probably live under laws that require cab drivers to be licensed and to charge a certain prescribed rate. But if you think those laws are there to protect you, think again. The licensing requirement tends to keep prices higher by limiting the number of cabs. In addition, minimum price rules tend to reduce price competition by existing drivers. Consumers lose both ways: It's harder to catch a cab, and we have to pay more when we're lucky enough to catch one.

Do these laws exist to benefit the cabbies, then? Hardly! Very few cab drivers have anything like the capital necessary to buy a cab medallion in a major city. (It's up to $600,000 per cab in New York City, according to Timothy Sandefur's recent book, *The Right to Earn a Living*.) So instead, a few large companies buy as many medallions as possible and lease them out to drivers at rents that may require a relatively poor driver to work the first five days of the week just to cover the lease payment for the medallion. Who wins? The big companies that have the capital to buy medallions, of course. The government's involvement doesn't counterbalance economic power; it creates it. And once government comes down on the side of restricting competition, we shouldn't be surprised to find stories like the 2010 story from Quincy, Illinois, where officials arrested a guy for giving drunks free rides home. They actually set up a sting to catch that guy!

Other types of government regulation work in much the same way. We touched on the problem of "regulatory capture" in an earlier essay on environmental regulations. In other realms as well, Big Business and Big Labor routinely tell Big Government what the regulations should say. And when Big Government comes through for them, they reward the compliant officials by making sure they get re-elected.

This is not an accusation of graft or even bad faith; it's just what happens once we accept the idea that government should intervene to change free-market outcomes. Regulation is costly, so businesses hire lobbyists to minimize the regulatory burdens that fall on them. The overhead costs of employing so many lobbyists are much easier for big companies to bear, so they typically wind up hiring the sharpest lawyers and spending the most money on lobbying efforts. And once they attain that favored insider status, the temptation to use it against their competitors is hard to resist. In this way, government ends up magnifying the dominance of the biggest businesses instead of neutralizing it.

Writing in the Cato Policy Report in 2010, Tim Carney gave a modern example from the running shoe industry. It seems that Nike left the Board of Directors of the Chamber of Commerce because Nike wanted government to regulate greenhouse gases; this was taken in some quarters as a sign of high-mindedness by Nike. But in fact, it was easy for Nike to support domestic greenhouse gas regulations because *Nike makes its shoes in Asia*. But New Balance, Nike's smaller competitor, makes its shoes in New England. Nike's support of regulatory burdens for shoe manufacturers would actually *help* Nike because it would significantly raise its domestic rival's costs.

At a 2010 candidate forum in Silver Spring, someone asked candidates for county council to summarize all the steps he would have to take in order to start operating a food truck selling Jamaican food. One staffer responded that the first thing to get straight was that it was going to take a long time to get the necessary approvals. An incumbent councilman then explained that the county would not be able to license the truck for operation near an existing Jamaican restaurant because that would raise "competition issues." When a challenger for office observed that it's no wonder people don't start more small businesses in Montgomery County, he was shouted down by the other incumbents, who rallied around this nakedly protectionist regulatory scheme.

It's worth recalling that we find ourselves here on Earth under circumstances that require us to work to feed ourselves. We have material needs, and we satisfy them through economic activity. The person in Silver Spring who wants to earn a living selling Jamaican food is not asking for any special privilege that ought to require a government license; he is not asking government to *make* anyone buy food from him. He is asking only for a liberty he was born with, no matter where he was born: the liberty to supply something of value to his fellow citizens at a mutually agreeable price. When government attempts to revoke that liberty, it imposes a burden that falls heaviest precisely on the people who are most in need of economic opportunity. When a majority of us finally come to understand that, *and vote that way*, then—finally—the era of Big Government will truly be over.

What's Wrong with "Stimulus" Spending?

One of my best teachers admonishes me to do more than preach to the choir. Specifically, while many people already deplore the Bush-Obama bailouts and stimulus bills, there are others (including Paul Krugman and many of his *New York Times* readers) who still believe, or at least hope, that aggressive overspending will restore the economy to vigor. What can I say to stimulus supporters to change their minds?

I can't do justice to such a big question in a short essay for a general audience; for that the reader must consult the works of the many economists who do not share Professor Krugman's view of the world. Some of them, like F.A. Hayek and Milton Friedman, also have Nobels to their credit. They don't happen to write in the *New York Times*, which is a shame for all of us. But if you haven't read their views somewhere, you should seek them out.

I'll emphasize just two points here: First, we have evidence that stimulus policies are not working and have not worked in the past. And second, if we consult our own experience of what makes us spend or invest or hire, we see that heavy government involvement in the economy not only fails to "stimulate" much economic activity, it actually makes us less likely to take the kinds of actions that are necessary in order to get the economy back on track.

We've been allegedly "stimulating the economy" nonstop since 2002, through massive deficit spending and an unprecedented amount of easy money from the Federal Reserve which kept interest rates low despite the red ink. But the first overt "stimulus" bill that I recall in the current downturn was President Bush's $168 billion version in February 2008. This, you'll recall, was the program by which we borrowed money in order to mail ourselves checks and take ourselves out to dinner.

Next, skipping over a few smaller bailouts, we had the Bush administration's bank bailout bill of October 2008. For that, we authorized another $700 billion. In addition, many in Congress resisted a $700 billion bank bailout but signed on after it was linked to a $150 billion tax cut that passed at the same time.

Then we had the massive spending spree that the Obama administration packaged as the American Reinvestment and Recovery Act, for which we borrowed another $787 billion. And since then, smaller mini-binges for automakers, appliance manufacturers, etc., not to mention a payroll tax cut which, incredibly, reduces payments into the Social Security program just as the payouts were already beginning to exceed the revenues.

What have we stimulated? The empirical results are not entirely conclusive, but they certainly don't provide any basis for celebrating the stimulus as a great policy success. Unemployment is no longer at its post-2008 highs, but it is still higher than it was before we adopted these "stimulus" policies.

These results corroborate the experience we had with stimulus policies during the Great Depression. President Hoover tried everything to stimulate the economy from 1929 to 1932, but nothing worked. Even the unprecedented stimulus policies of FDR's New Deal didn't do the job. Not until after World War II—when government spending actually *fell precipitously* in 1945-47—did our economy get healthy again.

Even Japan's experience with stimulative fiscal policy gives us reason to doubt its effectiveness. As a group of 300 economists stated in a joint letter they signed in opposition to the first major Obama stimulus bill, "More government spending by Hoover and Roosevelt did not pull the United States economy out of the Great Depression in the 1930s. More government spending did not solve Japan's 'lost decade' in the 1990s. As such, it is a triumph of hope over experience to believe that more government spending will help the U.S. today. To improve the economy, policy makers should focus on reforms that remove impediments to work, saving, investment and production. Lower tax rates and a reduction in the burden of government are the best ways of using fiscal policy to boost growth."

But stimulus defenders, particularly those belonging to the Keynesian school, can make the (untestable) claim that things would have been worse without the stimulus spending; or that the reason earlier stimulus attempts failed was that they weren't big enough. That's pure ideology, but it's not impossible, so let's turn to a couple of important theoretical reasons for questioning the Keynesians' story.

People who aren't actually engaged in business often look at the economy as a collection of aggregate statistics like GDP and the unemployment rate. One of the most important steps one can make toward economic literacy is to recognize that those aggregate statistics are designed to *measure* real-world economic behavior like spending or hiring, rather than to affect it. Think: Do you make your purchasing decisions based on GDP or the unemployment rate? Or do you consult your personal circumstances? One of the central insights of libertarian economists is that no matter how many people's actions you're trying to examine, every single person in the group will act "at the micro level," that is, based on his or her own desires, resources, opportunities, and alternatives. We can't change what economic actors are doing just by goosing government statistics with extra spending. So while there is no question that government can *raise* GDP by spending money (because government spending is one component of GDP), it simply does not follow that raising GDP puts people back to work.

This focus on "the micro level" also helps highlight one of the most neglected shortcomings of stimulus spending, which is the appallingly low correlation between the recipients of federal dollars and the people those dollars are intended to help. In the standard account accepted uncritically by most cable news anchors, the government's direct expenditures on big infrastructure projects like bridges and high-speed rail will help put unemployed construction workers back to work. It takes less than a minute's reflection to see how silly this is. Stimulus proponents speak as if the announcement of a high-speed rail project will cause tens of thousands of unemployed carpenters to pick up their hammers (or nail guns), drive to the spot where the new rail line is supposed to start, and be at work the next day. But the reality is that these federal contracts will be put out for competing bids, and in virtually all cases those contracts will be won by bidders who are *already going concerns* with their own employees. Will they hire some carpenters? Maybe, but not necessarily, and in any event *most* of the stimulus will go to people who already have jobs. Politicians who focus on aggregates like GDP miss this crucial shortcoming of "stimulus" policies.

Then there's the uncertainty problem. New productive activity, like starting a business and hiring some people, occurs only when individuals can predict a good return on their investment. So imagine that you're a recently unemployed chef, and you're wondering whether to wait things out or use your savings to open a new restaurant. You know there's a lot of competition, but you're confident your food will be tastier than theirs. You also know that some people won't want to pay what you want to charge, but you realize you don't need to win every customer in order to succeed financially. Looking only at your potential customers and your potential competitors, you're convinced it's a good idea.

But there are other risks you can't evaluate as easily. You understand your taxes may go up at the end of this year, and your profit margins were already pretty tight to begin with. You may even get hit with a soda tax. You know your health insurance costs are going up, even if you don't understand when or how. You keep seeing horrifying charts of what the Federal Reserve is doing to the money supply, and you worry that once a recovery actually comes, inflation may make your costs rise uncontrollably. And you keep hearing that government might regulate the trans-fat content of the food you serve. Because these things are all controlled by government rather than by you or your customers or your employees, they're not only outside your control, they're beyond your power to predict. So you sit tight, because of what economists call "regime uncertainty."

In this environment, it could hardly matter less to you whether the government is or is not spending, say, another $26 billion to plug holes in municipal government budgets. You don't know how much of that money will come to your community, or what your municipal government will do with it, or what will happen next year if the funding isn't renewed by the next Congress. If the success of your restaurant depends on that, it's not a risk you're willing to take. It's a safe bet that lots of people will always like good food at a fair price, because they always have. But there's just no telling what Congress might do—particularly a Congress dumb enough to *borrow money to destroy cars,* as Congress did in the 2009 "cash for clunkers" program.

The government could try to stimulate the opening of restaurants with a new-restaurant-owner tax credit, and that might stimulate you. But then again it might not, because you're not going to open the restaurant at all if it's only profitable in year one when the government is subsidizing it. And in any event, the restaurant stimulus bill isn't going to create any more certainty for your neighbor who is wondering whether to hire another salesperson at his bookstore. On the contrary, the more the government meddles, the less attractive *most* private investments become.

Stimulus spending is not entirely without effect, of course. If you happen to run a business that supplies what the government is buying, you'll profit handsomely. (Our recent fiscal and monetary policies have been very good for banks, for example.) But the people who take in all the hot money aren't as dumb as Congress seems to be hoping. They know the sudden increase in the demand for their services is artificial, and they know the government can't keep spending this way forever. So they're unlikely to change their behavior very much based on something they expect to be a one-time windfall. They're more likely to salt the money away for the rainy day they have every reason to expect soon. And that's one reason why banks, who are supposed to be in the business of lending money, have not been lending money.

Many 8th District voters know exactly what I'm talking about. A lot of us have done very well as a result of the increasing concentration of power and money in Washington. But it's bad for the country, and ultimately nothing that is bad for the country can possibly be good for the Washington suburbs. Not in the long run, anyway. And with our national debt approaching $16 trillion, our unfunded future debts above $118 trillion, and both numbers rising briskly, the "long run" may be shorter than we think.

Libertarianism and the Poor

We know free markets produce more prosperity, and we know government spending is often ineffective or worse. But many are nonetheless reluctant to embrace libertarian ideas because of their commitment to social justice. Without the welfare state, how would Libertarians take care of the poor?

The short answer is: Voluntarily. Libertarians know as well as anyone else that many people in our society sometimes find themselves in difficult circumstances through no fault of their own. We are as likely as anyone else to believe that looking out for the least fortunate among us is not only compassionate but essential to a healthy community. And many of us, including this writer, come from religious traditions that leave no room for doubt about the obligation to help the poor. For most of us, then, the question is not *whether* to help the poor, but *how*. And our historical experience strongly suggests that government programs just don't improve the welfare of the poor as well as voluntary assistance does.

The first problem with government aid is that it is easily misdirected. Government anti-poverty programs may be intended as boons for the poor, but they tend to become boondoggles for the powerful. This shouldn't surprise us, because when we make charity part of a government budget we inevitably place it in competition with other budgetary priorities. In a politically driven process, if it's the nameless needy versus failed Wall Street banks, the needy don't stand a chance. The working poor would have a much better chance of getting ahead if they were simply permitted to keep more of what they produce.

In this country, at this very moment, there are working men and women who are too poor to afford their own homes, yet their taxes subsidize jumbo mortgages on beachfront mansions because of the mortgage-interest deduction Congress wrote into our tax code. In this country, at this very moment, there are working men and women whose recent investment losses have forced them to postpone retirement, yet their taxes go to fund salaries, bonuses, and pensions for high-paid executives whom the government has chosen to relieve from any responsibility for running their businesses into the ground. These redistributions from the working poor to the networking rich don't comport with too many people's idea of social justice, but they are precisely the results we should by now expect from a system that countenances the redistribution of wealth according to the dictates of the politically powerful.

But can we rely on the voluntary alternative to fill the need? Will we keep giving if we're not forced to? Experience says yes. Experience teaches us that free people not only create abundance, they share it.

Aid works best when there are strong personal ties. While government entitlements all too often have the effect of perpetuating poverty, anyone who has ever leaned on a friend or a family member during hard times knows first-hand of the powerful bonds created by such mutual aid. It is altogether different from receiving an "entitlement" for which one has arguably "prepaid" with tax dollars. And the effect is usually personally trans-forming for both giver and receiver, in a way that bureaucratic transactions never can be. Strong families operate this way; they are strong not because the government requires it, but because family members spontaneously look out for each other and help each other thrive. Healthy neighborhoods operate on the same principle.

But the flourishing of global organizations like Save the Children, the Red Cross, and Doctors Without Borders dem-onstrates how well voluntary charity can work even when per-sonal connections are remote or non-existent and geographic distances are vast. We give voluntarily to the victims of hur-ricanes, earthquakes, and tsunamis. Humans empathize, and empathy works.

Then there is the layer between the neighborhood and the large non-profit—the space we refer to as "civil society." As David Boaz describes in his book, *Libertarianism: A Primer*, the "ales" of medieval and early modern England brought communities together "for drinking, dancing, and games, paying above-mar-ket prices to help out a neighbor: church-ales, to raise money for the parish; bride-ales, to get a marrying couple started; and help-ales, to assist those who had fallen on hard times." One sees in these customs the same instinct toward mutual aid that now survives in institutions from bake sales to church bingo to black-tie fundraising galas. We find parallel traditions in many different African, Asian, and Latin American cultures, going by names like *susu, hui, keh,* or *tanda.*

Fraternal societies such as the Masons, Elks, Odd Fellows, and Knights of Pythias are also the descendants of a venerable tradi-tion of mutual aid. Historically, such fraternal and "friendly" societies distinguished themselves sharply from "charity," as they were based on relationships among equals with the com-mon desire to help each other through sickness, old age, and hard times. This element of relationship bound the participants together more tightly in community, and encouraged responsible behavior by the recipients of aid—precisely what cannot happen under a system of legal entitlements.

Given all this history, the idea that people are insufficiently generous and that redistribution of wealth must therefore be required by law must be one of the most extensively falsified theories in all of political thought. And on reflection, it's quite odd to think that people acting on their own, with money they personally control, would be *less* willing to give generously than they are when they act through their legislative representatives. People typically give *more* when they have more say in making sure their donation will not be wasted.

Unfortunately, big government is slowly "squeezing out" these older and better ways of voluntarily helping the poor. That's bad for the poor, because government programs don't work as well. But it's also bad for the rest of us, because it impoverishes that important layer of civil society in which people of different races, religions, and political beliefs come together to celebrate their common humanity. It's good for Republicans and Democrats to work together at Habitat for Humanity. It's good for Jews and Muslims to serve together on the board of the local AIDS clinic. These voluntary associations are ostensibly for limited charitable purposes, but they make us stronger in rich and subtle ways. We need to reverse the tendency of big government to suffocate this layer of civil society.

Thus, the Libertarian approach to helping the poor is superior to the big-government approach on two counts. It is superior because private organizations—both for-profit and not-for-profit—can take care of the poor more effectively than any government program. And it is superior because a Libertarian approach to politics strengthens the layer of civil society that performs this and many other important social functions without the necessity of government involvement.

But don't take my word for it. Instead, consult your own common sense. Imagine that you have entered and won an essay contest on the plight of the world's poor. You wrote an extremely compassionate and well-argued essay, citing holy scripture from several world religions as well as pagan philosophers throughout recorded history. As the winner of the contest, you are now permitted to direct the spending of a $10 million fund for the alleviation of suffering among the poorest and most vulnerable among us. As you begin to think in earnest about how to distribute the $10 million, you have many worthy charities to consider: from the local soup kitchen in a neighborhood church basement all the way to the Gates Foundation or the Red Cross. Go ahead and think of one or two before you continue reading.

Done? Do you have your top choice or two?

Now, did it occur to you, for even a moment, to give that $10 million to the U.S. Department of Health and Human Services or the U.S. Department of Agriculture?

If not, then perhaps you should stop voting for people who think your tax dollars should be spent that way.

There's No Such Thing as a Free Colonoscopy

"Politics," said Groucho Marx, "is the art of looking for trouble, finding it everywhere, diagnosing it incorrectly, and applying the wrong remedies." It's hard to think of anything that illustrates this definition better than the 2010 "Patient Protection and Affordable Care Act," informally known as "Obamacare." No matter what the Supreme Court says about the constitutionality of the legislation, Congress should repeal it and start trying to undo some of the harm excessive government interference has already caused in health care markets.

The most basic problem with Obamacare is the idea that we can make health *care* more affordable by expanding the availability of health *insurance*. This shows a complete misunderstanding of how insurance works and what it can and can't do.

Insurance is a way of protecting against catastrophic risks, not a way of financing purchases you are almost certain to make. For example, most people who own their homes buy fire insurance, because they would be wiped out if fire destroyed what is probably their most valuable single asset. The cost of fire insurance is low relative to the potential loss from a fire, because very few homes actually get destroyed by fire or flood or anything else in any given year. The risk-spreading makes it a good deal, because it converts the risk of a catastrophic loss you cannot afford into a relatively minor expense of homeownership that you can afford.

In addition, real insurance can sometimes have the effect of reducing the chance that the insured risk will occur. For example, when insurance companies give people discounts for smoke alarms, smoke alarm usage tends to increase, and losses from fires tend to decrease. Good underwriting prices the risk accurately and encourages people to try harder to avoid losses.

Insurance is not magic, however. For one thing, it's not free; insurance companies have to collect more in premiums than they actually pay out in claims, and they have to collect *enough* more that they can pay their employees and still show a profit for their shareholders. In addition, there are certain things real insurance does not cover. Homeowner's insurance doesn't cover purely elective expenses, like the cost of installing new outdoor lighting or renovating a kitchen. It also doesn't cover routine maintenance expenses, like the cost of painting the outside or trimming nearby trees or cleaning the gutters—notwithstanding the fact that these are very important things to do for the long-term preservation of the house.

And importantly, even if homeowner's insurance did cover the cost of annual gutter cleaning, that really wouldn't do anyone any good because it doesn't involve any real risk-spreading. If 100 homeowners who used to hire gutter cleaners directly decide instead to take out insurance policies that cover gutter cleaning, the total cost goes up (because the insurance company has to pay its employees too), with no corresponding benefit to the homeowners. (There may be a *huge* benefit to the insurers—which perhaps suggests how Obamacare got through Congress.)

For many years, health insurance has become more and more like my imaginary gutter-cleaning insurance, and not nearly enough like real-life homeowner's insurance. Most health insurance plans do cover the risk of catastrophic injury or chronic illness, and I suspect that's the most important reason people want health insurance. But they also cover elective procedures and routine maintenance, and in fact most plans cover routine checkups *preferentially*. But because insurance companies charge between $1.30 and $1.50 in premiums for every dollar of benefits, the effect of throwing such routine procedures into the pool is to raise costs substantially. And it's this feature of health "insurance" that makes it so expensive and makes healthy young people want to opt out of it.

The reason many young people do *not* opt out, and didn't even before Obamacare, is because frequently someone else pays for the insurance policy. In this country, that someone is usually an employer (at least until the patient reaches age 65). And when an employer pays for the premium, then of course the insurance *does* make the worker better off, not because of risk-spreading but because of *cost-shifting*. And this is the second-most harmful feature of our current system of employer-sponsored over-insurance: it doesn't bring costs down; it just shifts them to whoever pays the premiums.

So our current approach to health care is based on two main principles: covering as much as possible (instead of just serious injuries and illnesses), and shifting the costs to people other than the patients (employers for some, taxpayers for others). This is definitely the wrong medicine.

When we make employers or taxpayers pay for "insurance" that covers nearly everything, we create the illusion that an extremely wide range of health care services are "free" (or substantially so) to everyone who has the "insurance." Of course, the services are not free; they're merely *pre-paid* by whoever pays the insurance premiums. But because the *patients* don't have to pay for them, many will undergo elective and routine procedures whether they need them or not. Over time this drives costs up by driving up total consumption of health care services.

It also drives *prices* up because it eliminates any market-based check on rising prices. If patients paid their own medical bills, rising prices would cure themselves, by discouraging unnecessary consumption and by stimulating competition among providers. But with health "insurance" as we know it, the signal sent by those rising prices never makes it back to the patient who's in charge of how much routine and elective care to consume: The cost of the procedure is paid by the insurance company rather than the patient. That makes premiums go up, but even the premium is paid by the patient's employer (or the taxpayers) rather than the patient. Goodbye price discipline.

Less tangibly, kitchen-sink health plans further expand our ever-more-expansive expectations of what "basic health care" entails, a fact that makes comparisons to other countries' experience less relevant. In a 2009 Bloomberg podcast, Princeton's Uwe Reinhardt, a leading authority on health care economics, tells the story of a Harvard Medical School professor whose mother in Florida told him she needed another MRI. The son replied skeptically, reminding her that she'd had an MRI only the month before. "Yeah," said the woman, "but I felt so good afterwards." There's no such thing as a free colonoscopy, but on the whole we are shockingly stupid consumers of health care because we have no incentive to be smart about it.

So why do we pay too much for health care? Precisely because we "insure" it so prodigiously. The way to save money would be to use less and pay only for what we use, instead of buying too much on a pre-paid basis and then treating it like a public good.

But aren't insurance markets private? Why doesn't private enterprise come up with a better alternative? I'll try to answer that question in my next essay.

How Government Drives Up Health Costs

In my last essay, I explained that "health insurance" as we know it raises health care costs by encouraging over-consumption, eliminating the price discipline we would see if patients paid their own costs, and making patients progressively dumber about the costs and benefits of their treatment. These effects flow primarily from the twin pillars of our modern health insurance market: coverage of nearly everything, and payment by somebody other than the patient (usually an employer or a government program).

The question a Libertarian should answer is: Why hasn't the private market developed in such a way as to give us a better alternative? And the answer is: Because the government has deliberately steered the market toward what we have today.

The association of health "insurance" with full-time employment began in the 1940s, when FDR's wage and price controls forbade employers from raising wages to attract workers during the wartime economy. Unable to raise wages, employers began adding benefits (which they were allowed to do), including health insurance. Somewhat paradoxically, the part of the government paying attention to the labor movement ruled in 1945 and 1949 that health benefits could not be reduced in the middle of a labor contract, and that such benefits should be considered part of the wage package during collective bargaining with unions.

The federal government thus created a policy framework that could ratchet up health benefits when the labor market was tight, while at the same time making it very hard for employers to make health benefits less generous. That cemented the employment-health insurance connection. Writing in the *New England Journal of Medicine,* David Blumenthal notes, "Between 1940 and 1950, the number of persons enrolled in private health plans increased from 20.6 million to 142.3 million . . . . By 1948, when President Harry S. Truman decided to advocate again for national health insurance, private health insurance was an established fact of life that not only had diminished the apparent need for government action but also had spawned a strong, new insurance industry with a stake in the status quo."

But why do employers choose policies that insure routine services instead of just the treatment of serious illnesses and injuries? That has government's fingerprints all over it as well. In 1954, the IRS declared that health insurance premiums paid by employers should *not* be taxed as income to the workers. This tax loophole has fueled the huge cost-shifting trend that discourages careful consumption and creates the illusion that health care is "free." Largely as a result of this one loophole, out-of-pocket spending by consumers of health care in the United States fell from 48 percent of all health care costs in 1960 to just 15 percent in 2000.

In addition, according to the National Association of Health Underwriters, more than 1,000 governmental mandates for "free" medical services were already in existence even before Obamacare, and the NAHU attributed up to 25% of premiums to these (unfunded) mandates. Sometimes governments require coverage of particular procedures or diagnostic tools; sometimes they require that plans cover certain classes of alternative therapies, like acupuncture or massage therapy. Not only do these mandates exacerbate the over-consumption and price-insensitivity we looked at in the last essay, they also have the practical effect of forcing insurance companies to sell different policies in different states, thus limiting competition among insurers. Thus, while some "reform" proponents rail against the evil insurance companies for coming between patients and their doctors, the reality is that state governments have been calling the tunes (without paying the piper) to a remarkable and regrettable degree *for years*.

This is, then, another case in which years of uncoordinated government interventions have created a distorted incentive structure, producing disastrous unintended consequences. Business executive David Goldhill, in an excellent 2009 article in *The Atlantic*, makes a nice point about the parallels between the housing bubble and the health care problem:

> The housing bubble offers some important lessons for health-care policy. The claim that something— whether housing or health care—is an undersupplied social good is commonly used to justify government intervention, and policy makers have long striven to make housing more affordable. But by making housing investments eligible for special tax benefits and subsidized borrowing rates, the government has stimulated not only the construction of more houses but also the willingness of people to borrow and spend more on houses than they otherwise would have. . . .
>
> As with housing, directing so much of society's resources to health care is stimulating the provision of vastly more care. Along the way, it's also distorting

demand, raising prices, and making us all poorer by crowding out other, possibly more beneficial, uses for the resources now air-dropped onto the island of health care. Why do we view health care as disconnected from everything else? Why do we spend so much on it? And why, ultimately, do we get such inconsistent results? Any discussion of the ills within the system must begin with a hard look at the tax-advantaged comprehensive-insurance industry at its center.

So, in a nutshell, the major problems with health "insurance" today—its overly comprehensive scope, its high cost, and its dependence on employment—grew out of specific government policies with huge unintended consequences. This means, at a minimum, that we ought not to base support for a government-centered reform effort on the facile supposition that "it can't get any worse than what the insurance companies have given us." Indeed, I think we should draw the further conclusion that government interventions have already made this problem far worse than it needed to be, and even the most fervent supporters of greater government involvement should have the humblest of expectations about our ability to improve on the overall effect of so many billions of individual decisions.

Can we do anything to help now? Yes, but only if we embrace what works: Liberty. I'll say more about that in the third essay in this series.

Health Care Freedom, Not "Free" Health Care

At the risk of wildly oversimplifying, my last two essays have argued that health insurance stinks and it's mostly the government's fault. It's time for us to recognize that our national health care debate is fundamentally a problem of resource distribution. We have plenty of health care resources, but some people overuse them and some people can't get to them at all. So what we really need is a system that efficiently directs resources to the points at which the need for them is the greatest. Free markets do this better than any other method known to humankind.

This may sound radical, but . . . What if patients hired doctors and paid them directly? Some people might pay for checkups and treatments *a la carte*, while others might want to obtain services on a prepaid basis. There might even be privately managed membership organizations dedicated to improving their members' health—like HMOs, only they would actually need to keep their members happy and their costs as low as possible because the bills would be paid by the patients rather than their employers or the taxpayers. Can anyone honestly doubt that this sort of system would spawn innovations that no one reading this essay has thought of?

Could people pay for such expensive treatments directly? For the most part, yes. The expenses are large, but almost never larger than the price of a new television, let alone a new or even a used car. Somehow, virtually every household in the United States manages to finance these things without "insurance." And the price system somehow manages to put televisions into many households that are well below the poverty level. Of course, no one would want to be ruined by catastrophic or chronic illness, so people of all walks of life would want to purchase insurance against the risks they truly could not bear.

The real question is not whether people *could* pay directly for health care, but whether they *would*. And the obvious answer is, sometimes yes, sometimes no, depending on whether the *price* of any given treatment is less than or greater than its *value*. That's the secret ingredient that makes it all work, and that's the very thing our current system of *faux* insurance eliminates almost completely.

Here are the specific steps Congress should take to try to spark a free-market revolution within the government-dominated health-care sector we know today:

First, end unfunded coverage mandates at the federal level and pre-empt them at the state and local levels. I don't pretend to know how often women should have mammograms or when prostate screening should start, but the odds are overwhelmingly against anyone in my federal or state legislature having a better-informed opinion on those questions than a doctor and patient will arrive at together. Ending these mandates will allow people to buy insurance for the serious risks they can't afford, without being forced to pay for the health-care equivalent of a homeowner's policy that covers gutter cleaning.

Second, eliminate the preferential tax treatment for employer-sponsored health benefits as income to the covered employees. I'm generally anti-tax, but I'm even more anti-loophole, particularly when the loophole in question introduces a huge distortion into the way a sixth of our economy functions. Until we get rid of the tax subsidy for employer-sponsored health plans, the private employers who currently provide coverage for the majority of us will have little incentive to demand real insurance rather than the pre-paid medical services contracts that essentially buy us all kinds of stuff we don't need or want.

Third, mandate portability without respect to pre-existing conditions. Wait, did I just say "mandate"? Yes, but only for ten years—long enough to counteract the decades of government-induced linkage between health insurance and employment. Once the tax loophole for employer-sponsored health plans is eliminated, workers will increasingly opt for higher wages and the right to choose their own health coverage. Insurers will be happy to provide portability to these workers at a competitive price, and price competition will be stronger when the customer and the patient are one and the same.

Fourth, help the poor directly. As a Christian, I believe we should help the poor obtain health care, for the same reasons and in the same way that we help the poor obtain food and shelter. As a Libertarian, I believe we should do this through private charity, as we have since the dawn of health care. But even if government insists on replacing private charity with an entitlement program, that program should be focused on the financial needs of the very poor; it should not be a complete takeover of the entire health care industry. Voluntary transactions between doctors and patients must form the core of the health care system if we want it to function well.

Fifth, leave it alone. Health insurance has been such a popular subject of legislative fidgeting for the past twenty years that some promising reform ideas made it into law but never really had a chance to work before people were chatting up the Next Big Thing. People can't make rational decisions about things that are treated as perennial political footballs. In other words, Congress: It may itch while it heals, but don't scratch it.

Is any of this likely? Not unless we elect Libertarians to Congress. Fortunately, we can do that whenever we're ready for a new approach.

Downsizing D.C.

For those that aren't familiar with it, DownsizeDC.org is a great website to visit and a great organization to support. Their particular excellence, it seems to me, is their ability to translate libertarian ideals into concrete pieces of legislation that would improve the way Congress operates. Here, for example, are the six pieces of legislation they have highlighted for their "Downsize DC Agenda":

- *The "Read the Bills Act"*: The "Read the Bills Act," or RTBA, would require all bills to be posted on the Internet for seven days prior to any vote so that citizens could weigh in on the proposed text. The bills would also have to be read orally in the presence of a quorum in the House and the Senate. Perhaps more importantly, however, the RTBA would require all members of Congress who intend to vote in favor of any bill to file affidavits certifying that they had actually read it themselves and knew its contents. This would promote public participation in the legislative process, prevent legislators from explaining away votes for unpopular measures with the claim that they didn't know all the details in the bill, and—just maybe—discourage

Congress from writing bills that run to hundreds and even thousands of pages in order to regulate so many unnecessary details of our lives.

- *The "One Subject at a Time Act"*: This bill takes aim at a major reason for the existence of so many deeply unpopular laws: the propensity of Congress to bury a few unrelated special favors in the middle of a bill that is supposed to deal with something else entirely. The OSTA would require all bills to address only one subject. Furthermore, all bills would be required to carry a title that describes what is actually in the bill, rather than a misleading, propagandistic title like "PATRIOT Act" or "DISCLOSE Act."

- *The "Write the Laws Act"*: The WTLA attempts to end Congress's abdication of its constitutional power to decide what the laws are. In recent years, as evidenced by the recent financial "reform" bill, Congress has passed laws that are little more than general statements of policy accompanied by instructions to various regulatory agencies to write the substantive rules Congress couldn't be bothered with. This results, necessarily, in government by unelected bureaucrats and unelected judges. It also, quite often, produces the disgraceful spectacle of a Congress that agrees to have a federal law about something without agreeing on what the federal law should say.

- *The "Free Competition in Currency Act"*: Those who are only beginning to learn about libertarianism may be puzzled by the inclusion of this bill, but it addresses one of the most fundamental economic problems we have: the corrosive influence of the Federal Reserve's easy-money policies. Those policies facilitate excessive spending and unnecessary wars by Congress, and are the major cause of economic "bubbles" that wreak so much havoc on our prosperity. The FCCA would end government or quasi-government monopolies on the issuance of coins or currency, so that people would be free to deal in money that could not be arbitrarily drained of its value by government fiat. Although the concept of competing forms of money may be strange to most Americans today, it has been the norm for most of our history as a nation. Historically, and across many different civilizations, gold, silver, and other precious metals have been the commodities used most frequently and most successfully as money, and so the FCCA also prohibits capital gains taxation of transactions in these metals, in order to prevent the government from making them less competitive forms of money in the future. (Readers who want to learn more about these issues should read Downsize DC.org's FCCA background page, and may also wish to read Murray Rothbard's excellent introduction to the problem, *What Has Government Done to Our Money?*)

- *The "Enumerated Powers Act"*: "This one is easy. It requires Congress to specify in each bill precisely which enumerated Constitutional power it is exercising. The point, of course, is that there are really not very many enumerated powers that the Constitution gives to Congress. Bank bailouts, gun laws, drug laws, farm subsidies, automobile manufacturing, and free colonoscopies are just some of the many things our founders never intended Congress to have anything to do with. The Enumerated Powers Act would not prevent Congress from twisting and stretching the words of Article I, Section 8 of our Constitution in order to justify all manner of meddling, but it would make members of Congress go on the record with their tortured interpretations so that voters could hold them properly accountable.

- *The "Fiscal Responsibility Act"*: This one is easy, too. It cuts Congressional pay for every year the budget remains in deficit. A one-year deficit costs each member of Congress

5% of his pay. If deficits last for two or more years, the annual cut becomes 10%. Pay is restored to pre-deficit levels only after the budget is restored to balance.

I also favor some broader reform measures designed to improve Congress's performance, including fundamental tax reform, term limits, and redistricting reform. But I applaud DownsizeDC.org's efforts to focus on these six specific pieces of legislation, and I support them all.

What About Global Warming?

In an earlier essay, we talked about the libertarian approach to environmental protection, which emphasizes the ways in which property rights harmonize economic and environmental interests, as well as the ability of the judicial system to vindicate each landowner's right to prevent environmental damage to his or her own property. But some have pointed out that this approach works far less well with air pollution than with other kinds of environmental problems—which is true. And others, citing what may be the biggest air pollution problem of all, have asked, "What about global warming?"

I'm not qualified to offer any reliable opinions about the science here, *i.e.,* about whether the Earth is still getting warmer, or whether the warming has peaked and we are now in a cooling trend. I consider myself neither a "denier" nor an "alarmist." There is no reason anyone should care about my opinions on the various scientific theories we all read. But for those who nonetheless want to know:

- We know the climate is constantly changing. We know it moves in both directions, and so far it has never failed to reverse direction after some period of time. In other words, it has never yet reached an irreversible tipping point.

- Scientists in the very recent past have been surprised by the direction in which global temperatures move. We know this from all the "global cooling" predictions that were in fashion until just before the "global warming" predictions started; and perhaps also from the recent shift in vocabulary away from "global warming" and toward the less specific (and therefore unfalsifiable) "climate change."

- I think we do not yet understand the many different causes of climate change, or their apparent cyclicality, well enough to place any confidence at all in long-term temperature predictions, particularly predictions based on models that have already proven unreliable over periods far shorter than the ones we're trying to model.

But there's nothing distinctively Libertarian about those opinions. What *is* distinctively Libertarian is my belief that, *even if we had better predictive models of all the non-human elements, and even if those models unambiguously pointed to significant human causation of sustained global warming,* the climate change pessimists would still be making at least two big mistakes. First, they seem to ignore human adaptability, which makes it rash to project the continuation of any catastrophic trend over a period as long as 100 years or more. And second, they uncritically endorse coordinated government action, rather than decentralized innovation, as the best strategy for averting future harms.

The role of human adaptability is perhaps best illustrated by The Great Horse-Manure Crisis of 1894. In case your history teacher skipped that chapter, the story has been charmingly told by Stephen Davies in an essay for *The Freeman.* The short version is that London, New York, and other great cities of the 1890s were growing so rapidly that the sheer number of horses

was becoming a problem—a very smelly and unsightly problem. As Davies writes,

> The larger and richer that cities became, the more
> horses they needed to function. The more horses, the
> more manure. Writing in the *Times* of London in 1894,
> one writer estimated that in 50 years every street in
> London would be buried under nine feet of manure.
> Moreover, all these horses had to be stabled, which used
> up ever-larger areas of increasingly valuable land. And
> as the number of horses grew, ever-more land had to
> be devoted to producing hay to feed them (rather than
> producing food for people), and this had to be brought
> into cities and distributed—by horse-drawn vehicles.
> It seemed that urban civilization was doomed."

We know how this story ends, of course, so it is easy for us to
poke fun at the 1894 forecast. But the problem was taken quite
seriously at the time. In fact, in 1898 an international urban-
planning conference in New York was *abandoned* after only
three of the ten days originally scheduled, "because none of the
delegates could see any solution to the growing crisis posed by
urban horses and their output." What happened, of course, was
innovation; the appearance of a new technology that changed
everything.

This has happened throughout our history. In Matt Ridley's
excellent book, *The Rational Optimist*, he recounts how Thomas
Robert Malthus famously predicted in 1798 that food supply
could never keep pace with population because there must be a
limit to the productivity of agricultural land. That doom was
averted when new fertilizers came into use, made of enormous
deposits of nitrogen-rich bird droppings on various islands.
These were extensively "guano-mined" for fertilizer throughout the 19th century, until a new crisis appeared on the horizon: The guano supply would soon be exhausted, and by 1898

an eminent British chemist was warning that "all civilisations stand in deadly peril of not having enough to eat" unless more nitrogen could be found. Within fifteen years, Fritz Haber and Carl Bosch had invented a way to make large quantities of inorganic nitrogen fertilizer from steam, methane, and air. Crisis averted once again.

The point is not that we shouldn't worry about climate change, or peak oil, or bird flu, or whatever; sometimes (but only sometimes) the innovators who falsify such prophecies of doom make their breakthroughs precisely because they are worried. The point is rather that even if all the climate models were entirely correct, it would be beyond ridiculous to assume that the next 100 years will bring no improvements in energy efficiency, no increases in agricultural productivity, none of the customary dips in birth rates that we usually see with economic development——in short, none of the innovation that has constantly characterized human existence since men made axes out of stones. I may not know what *will* happen over the next 100 years, but a century of total stagnation certainly will *not* happen.

How about the pessimists' second mistake, their trust in coordinated government action? In many ways, this is but another lesson from the same set of historical examples. Revolutionary improvements in our living standards are revolutionary precisely because they are unexpected. Even when they are consciously sought after by many people at once (which is by no means all of the time), success generally comes from diversity of effort, with many people working independently or in small groups, each with a somewhat different approach. We try many things because no one knows for sure what will work. (Think: If we *did* know what would work, no one would be warning of crisis!)

Thus, if we knew for a fact that carbon dioxide emissions were raising our planet's temperature by ten degrees per century (much more than the pessimists predict), and that the *only possible* solution was to reduce the carbon footprint of all existing methods of transportation, manufacturing, and agriculture, coordinated multilateral government action would *still* be a terrible idea. Indeed, there would be no surer way to seal our doom than to put a single multinational body in charge of decreeing a single approach to the problem. And that's no knock on the United Nations; *no one* is smart enough to make centrally planned action perform better than independent decision-making. It just doesn't happen. Unfortunately, people in government won't understand that point until we start voting as if we understand it ourselves.

We Can't Have Big Government *a la carte*

Even die-hard fans of Big Government usually admit that a wide range of federal programs are pointless or worse. But often I meet people who are so attached to some particular program that they cannot bring themselves to accept any political philosophy that might lead to less money for their favorite. Almost everyone, including me, can find something in a $3.8 trillion budget that is personally appealing even though it can't be justified on libertarian principles like the non-aggression principle. Whether it's environmental regulations or high-speed rail or NASA or foreign aid, these people essentially ask: Can't we embrace the benefits of small government generally, but make an exception for *my* pet program?

This sounds theoretically possible, but I think our experience justifies us in saying it is not. Big Government seems not to be available *a la carte*. We have to take the bad with the good. And that means that if the choice between private action and government program is at all close, we ought to have a very strong bias for the private option. Because the pet programs we can't justify as protections of our persons and property are almost never so great as to be worth the high social cost of a government that acts without strong limits.

It sounds pragmatic to make case-by-case determinations about federal programs instead of sticking to a strong limiting principle like the non-aggression principle. But the problem with *ad hoc* picking and choosing is that it makes members of Congress practically incapable of saying no to any significant constituency. It's very hard to bail out banks and then say no to automakers or local governments. It's very hard to explain why Congress should let the free market work in any sector unless Congress lets the free market work in every sector. And it's very hard to blow money on any program as idiotic as "cash for clunkers" and then say no to equally idiotic proposals like "cash for caulkers" or "cash for can-openers." The slope gets very slippery very fast, and we know that for a fact because we're currently sliding down it at breakneck speed.

Some people think there is no limiting principle; that it's OK to fund Big Government programs as long as they're popular. After all, if more than fifty percent of us want to support such programs, why shouldn't we? But it's a fantasy to think that Congress responds only to numerical majorities. Sugar quotas are demonstrably bad for nearly everyone who buys sugar—a very large majority, as political majorities go. Yet sugar quotas persist *precisely because* the group they benefit is so much smaller than the group they injure. It is the concentration of very large benefits for a very small number of sugar producers that makes the sugar producers willing to spend relatively large amounts of money lobbying for the quotas. And it is the wide spreading of the costs of the quotas (through higher sugar prices) that virtually eliminates any significant opposition to the quotas. This phenomenon repeats itself on page after page of the federal budget, and the only way for us to change it is to insist on a principled basis for rejecting all appeals for special treatment of this or that business or industry.

Paradoxically, the pick-and-choose approach leads to wasteful spending so consistently that we really ought to consider it an iron law of politics: *Once we move beyond the protection of persons and property, it is never possible to have the good spending without the bad.* If you vote to fund mental health programs at the National Institute of Mental Health, you will someday learn that NIMH spent $823,200 to teach uncircumcised African men how to wash their private parts. NIMH actually did that. If you're learning that now for the first time, you will be shocked, but you shouldn't be. Not anymore.

And it's not just the money, either; it's also the power. If you vote for a federal government that sets itself up in charge of our environmental choices, there will certainly come a day when you will find yourself swearing at a low-flush toilet that doesn't provide enough flush, or squinting beneath a compact fluorescent light bulb that doesn't provide enough light. The same bureaucrats whom you hire to do the environmental stuff you made an "exception" for won't be able to help themselves from doing all manner of other things that they just know are good for you. And now we've placed them in charge of our health care. How many times can they fool us with these "camel's nose" maneuvers before we get wise?

This principled approach for rejecting federal programs even when they are wildly popular parallels our traditional approach to civil liberties. We stand up for the free speech rights of some pretty repulsive characters because we know our own rights are measured by what we allow them to say. We don't let the sheriff beat confessions out of the guilty because we don't want him to beat confessions out of the innocent. We need to bring that kind of thinking to the task of setting our budget and policy priorities. We need to think harder about the terrible programs whenever we're debating a proposal we're tempted to like.

Fiscal Responsibility Now

It was August 3, 2010, at a candidate forum at Leisure World, when the man in the back of the room hit the nail on the head: Every candidate says it's very important for us to balance the federal budget, but they never give specifics. What, specifically, does each candidate propose to cut?

I gave a pretty specific answer that day, but it was nothing compared to the actual balanced budget proposal that Ohio Libertarian Travis Irvine and I released in October 2010. (An agency-level summary of the budget is reprinted as Appendix B; the contemporaneous press release is reprinted as Appendix A.) And the experience of producing a balanced budget helped me focus a bit more clearly on a few facets of the budget problem, and perhaps by extension the sorry state of our politics in general.

The fact that Travis and I were the only two candidates to produce a balanced federal budget for Fiscal Year 2012 spoke volumes about the people we currently have in Congress, and none of it is very flattering to them. Balancing the budget all in one year was very, very hard; it required deep cuts in spending

as well as the elimination of tax loopholes that many powerful people really like. But balancing the budget in two years
wouldn't have been that hard. Balancing the budget in four
years would have been *child's play*. So what are we to make of
people who produce ten-year budgets in which even the tenth
year fails to balance? We can only conclude that such people
do not really want to balance the budget. If they say they do,
they are lying. That's blunt language, but the conclusion is
inescapable.

This is a complete failure of nerve by the two major parties
rather than a question of gridlock. It's not as if we have a
Republican balanced budget plan on one side of the aisle and a
Democratic balanced budget plan on the other, with a lack of
national consensus about which one we should pass. No; we
have in fact *no proposal to balance the budget from either Democrats
or Republicans*, and most candidates won't even talk about their
future fiscal plans except in the vaguest and most general of
terms. Again, I think the only conclusion we can draw from
this is that the vast majority of politicians *in both major parties*
place their political careers above the health of the republic. By
contrast, Travis and I don't have political careers and we don't
particularly want them. We just want the government to run
right. So we tried to solve the problem everyone else was ignor-
ing: We crunched the numbers until our budget balanced. You
can decide for yourself what to do with the men and women
whose *job* was to do this but who nonetheless didn't even try. I
would recommend firing them.

Where do we go from here? Ultimately that's up to the voters.
I imagine voters will respond in one of two ways. One group
will look at our budget and say, "That's *all* you cut? Defense is
still too large, and I can't believe you're leaving Social Security
and Medicare untouched even temporarily. And where's the tax
reform?" This will be a small group, almost entirely composed
of Libertarians. But these are my people, and they are dear to

me; I value their good opinion, so I wish to say to them that some things take longer than one year. Because we took the need to balance the budget *in 2012* as an absolute constraint, we were unable to rely on many excellent policy proposals that we should absolutely try to implement as soon as possible. Tax reform, in particular, has long been at the top of my list.

By far the larger group of voters will look at the cuts we have proposed and they will be horrified. The ones who take the proposal seriously will call it Draconian, and perhaps a larger number will simply dismiss the proposal as unrealistic. This is the group I am most anxious to reach. I want to make them understand that the severity of the cuts we had to propose in order to achieve balance is a consequence of how far out of balance our budget currently is. It doesn't do us any good to propose "glide paths" or "sustainable trends" or other allegedly "moderate" solutions that aren't equal to size of the problem.

Our national debt and our future entitlement liabilities are already so high that we will not be able to repay additional loans we give ourselves from future income. Do you know what they call it when you take out a loan you know you can't repay? They call that stealing. We're stealing from the future right now, and the only fact that mitigates our guilt in any degree is that we aren't really stealing from our children anymore; we are so near the point of collapse right now that the vast majority of us will live to regret it if we don't step back from the brink.

Whichever group you fall into, take action. If you like the budget, tell your friends about it and urge as many candidates as possible to sign on. If you don't like our budget, ask your favored candidate what his or her alternative budget plan is. Now that we've shown that it *can be done*, you don't have to put up with any excuses any more. You sure don't have to put up with people who say it can't be done, or that it has to take ten years. That's unworthy of anyone's vote.

Let me end with an appeal to my fellow candidates, here in the 8th District and across the nation.

Each year's deficit adds to our debt burden, and we simply cannot afford any more debt unless we want to condemn ourselves and our children to sluggish economic growth, falling living standards, and increasing danger of financial collapse. We must break free from the swirling vortex of laziness, cowardice, and self-delusion that has prevented us from dealing with this problem. It's our job as candidates to propose ways to bring federal spending in line with federal revenues, in a way that respects individual liberty and makes us stronger as a nation and stronger in our local communities.

If you don't like our budget, do your own. You can get the agency budgets and historical figures from the Office of Management and Budget. You can find all kinds of great policy proposals from budget experts at Cato, Heritage, Brookings, and many other respectable think tanks. Use as much or as little of our budget as you want, and knock yourselves out. There are lots of different ways to balance the budget, and you might come up with something that even I like better.

But there's one thing you can't do with the budget any longer: You can't hide behind it. If you don't like our numbers, let's see yours. In particular, Chris Van Hollen, you've had a full-time job minding our money for ten years, and you've had all the resources of the Ways & Means Committee and the Budget Committee at your disposal. When are you going to balance the federal budget, and how?

Give Me Liberty

Let me ask you a very simple question: What color are yield signs?

Most people say yellow. I did.

But yield signs haven't been yellow in decades. Yield signs have now been red and white for about 40 years, which is more than twice as long as they were yellow. If you answered that yield signs are yellow today, you were letting some mental impression from long ago trump your more recent experience with yield signs. And unless you were driving back in the early 70s, your mental impression of the yellow yield sign may have been created by a toy or a picture rather than an actual yield sign; it may *never* have been true in your personal experience. If I asked you when you were looking at an actual yield sign, you wouldn't make that mistake.

Now suppose I ask you these questions: Which political party stands for limited government? Which political party stands for civil liberties? Which is the party of the free market? The party of peace?

It's important—critically important—for all of us to answer these questions based on our actual experience rather than the mental impressions we may have formed decades ago. If you want smaller government, vote Libertarian. If you want peace, vote Libertarian. If you want to restore free enterprise, vote Libertarian. If you cherish your right to freedom of speech, freedom of religion, and all the other precious civil liberties in our Bill of Rights, vote Libertarian. Voting for another party on false pretenses—or on reputations that haven't been accurate since your grandparents' day—won't get you what you want. It won't get you what you think you're voting for.

To my Republican friends in Maryland's 8ᵗʰ District: I know you are most anxious to stop the relentless growth of government. You want the budget to be balanced, and you want the regulatory burden on productive business enterprise to be cut back substantially. But I have bad news for you: The Republican party doesn't share your views. And even if it did, your party has been gerrymandered into impotence in this District. That doesn't mean you should give up and stay home, but it does mean that you should make sure your vote communicates what you really stand for. I've talked to enough of you to know that you don't really stand for the kind of government that Republican officeholders consistently favored over the last dozen years. Vote Republican, and you've successfully communicated only that you want John Boehner to lead the Congress. Vote Libertarian, and you've successfully communicated that you're for less government, more liberty, more prosperity, and more security.

To my Democratic friends in Maryland's 8ᵗʰ District: I know you are most anxious to make sure ordinary people have a fighting chance at economic security and personal liberty. You treasure your civil liberties and you're frustrated by all the money we waste on perpetual war. But I have bad news for you as well: Democrats are more like Republicans than you

162

think. The economic policies that Democrats have been pursuing may be good for the rich and powerful people who have made careers out of pretending to like the poor, but they do not actually make poor people richer. They make us all poorer, by squandering our resources and discouraging our innate drive to produce. The government powerful enough to do this to us has also continued to send our sons and daughters to fight and die in faraway places, and neither civil liberties nor the cause of peace has fared any better under Democrats than under Republicans. Tens of thousands of you know this, but you haven't been willing to criticize your own party for fear of sounding like the Republicans you despise. Beware! It was precisely that brand of party "loyalty" that allowed the Republican party of the Bush years to march over a cliff. Vote Democratic, and you've done your part to keep our country and your party barreling down the road to ruin. Vote Libertarian, and you've helped call all of us back to principles worthy of the party of Jefferson: less government, more liberty, more prosperity, and more security.

And what of my independent friends? Some of you are closet partisans, but surveys say about half of you are lifelong independents. And I know from talking to you that a good many of you are spitting mad at Democrats and Republicans alike. Some of you are so mad that you plan to stay home. Others plan to vote for the "lesser of two evils." For you, I have some good news: You don't have to do that anymore. And you shouldn't. After all, a twenty-foot ladder is no better than a ten-foot ladder if you're at the bottom of a fifty-foot hole. And unfortunately, that's where Democrats and Republicans have left us. We need to keep calling for that fifty-foot ladder until we get it, and we're fortunate that in our system we always get the kind of government we call for if we call persistently enough. This year, try calling for less government, more liberty, more prosperity, and more security.

There's a deeper problem with "lesser of two evils" voting: It's unworthy of our heritage, no matter what your party affiliation is. Our ancestors didn't fight and bleed for your rights to life, liberty, and the lesser of two evils. Patrick Henry did not thunder for all the ages, "Give me Liberty, or give me whatever everyone else is having." Martin Luther King did not stand on the steps of the Lincoln Memorial and tell us, "I have a dream, but I'll settle for less." No. The great ones who have preceded us showed their greatness in their commitment to principle— and specifically in their recognition that sometimes the "lesser of two evils" just isn't good enough.

Now it's your turn to march in that same parade of history. Don't blow it—your children are watching. Stand up and be counted for the kind of government you'd really like to have. Vote for less government, more liberty, more prosperity, and more security. Vote Libertarian.

Appendix A: Libertarian Candidates Release Balanced Federal Budget for 2012 (October 4, 2010 Press Release)

FOR IMMEDIATE RELEASE

4 October 2010

LIBERTARIAN CANDIDATES RELEASE BALANCED FEDERAL BUDGET FOR 2012

In an effort to give voters a real alternative to the big-spending politics of the Democratic and Republican parties, two Libertarian candidates for the U.S. House of Representatives have developed a federal budget that completely eliminates the federal budget deficit in one year.

Mark Grannis, the Libertarian candidate in Maryland's 8th District, teamed up with Travis Irvine, the Libertarian candidate in Ohio's 12th District, to produce the budget for fiscal year 2012 (the fiscal year that begins October 1, 2011, and the first fiscal year for which the next Congress will prepare a budget).

The Libertarian Balanced Federal Budget Proposal relies on a mix of spending cuts and revenue increases, though it increases revenue by eliminating tax loopholes rather than by changing tax rates. The proposal balances the budget despite keeping 2010 tax rates in place for all taxpayers.

The budget also proposes no changes to Social Security or Medicare, and only one relatively modest change to Medicaid: capping block grants to the states at 2010 funding levels and giving states greater responsibility for funding their Medicaid policy choices in the future. Grannis and Irvine both support more comprehensive entitlement reforms, but their aim was to show that the federal budget could be brought into balance without injecting those larger issues into the budget process.

Under the Libertarians' budget proposal, federal spending in 2012 would decline by $991 billion from the levels set forth in the President's 2011 Budget. The President's Budget requested total spending of $3,833,861,000,000 for 2011, a figure that remains only a request because Congress decided not to bother passing a 2011 budget. Under the Libertarian Balanced Federal Budget Proposal, spending would decline from $3.834 trillion to $2.843 trillion.

The President's 2011 Budget also included the Office of Management and Budget's estimate of what spending levels would look like for 2012. When compared to those levels rather than the 2011 levels, the Libertarian Balanced Federal Budget represents spending reductions of roughly $912 billion. The major spending cuts are described in the summary that accompanies this release, but some of the most significant items are:

- Spending cuts of <u>more than $150 billion in the Department of Defense</u>;

- Spending cuts of <u>more than $100 billion each in the Departments of Agriculture and Health and Human Services</u> ;

- Spending cuts of <u>more than $80 billion each in the Departments of Education and Transportation</u> (including elimination of the Department of Education);

- Spending cuts of <u>more than $40 billion each in the Departments of Housing and Urban Development</u> (which is also proposed for elimination) <u>and Transportation</u>;

- Meaningful cuts in every other federal agency, including <u>tens of billions of dollars each in the Departments of Energy, Homeland Security, Justice, Labor, and NASA.</u>

- Elimination of approximately <u>$20 billion in non-Medicaid block grants to state and local governments.</u>

- <u>Privatization of government programs</u> that previously cost over $26 billion, including Amtrak, the Postal Service, the Federal Aviation Administration, and the Transportation Safety Administration.

- An <u>end to the federal "War on Drugs,"</u> saving over $16 billion for the federal government and much more for state and local governments.

- Elimination of <u>"corporate welfare"</u> spending of over $12 billion; and

- A <u>5%, across-the-board spending cut</u> for all remaining federal spending.

On the revenue side, the Libertarians' budget proposal extends the tax rates currently in effect for all individuals regardless of income, but eliminates or phases out various tax credits, tax preferences, subsidies, and other loopholes worth more than $7 trillion over the next ten years. These tax gimmicks, known officially as "tax expenditures" because they benefit some people but not others in much the same way that government spending does, have grown significantly since 1986 and have recently been recognized as a major source of Washington's budget problem. Elimination of "tax expenditures" will generate approximately $414 billion in additional revenue in 2012, with the amount of additional revenue growing somewhat in later years.

Even with $1 trillion in spending cuts and more than $400 billion in new revenue from the elimination of "tax expenditures," the budget for fiscal year 2012 still would not balance without one last item: sale of approximately 22.5% of federal gold reserves. Grannis and Irvine propose to have the U.S. Mint sell half-ounce deficit-reduction coins to U.S. citizens in much the same way the government once sold war bonds. They project approximately $108 billion in additional 2012 revenue from this one-time sale of gold reserves. The $108 billion in revenue would be replaced in 2013 as the continued phase-out of certain tax expenditures generates additional revenue that could not be raised in 2012 without even more drastic budgetary changes.

In a video released to announce the budget, Grannis and Irvine invite other candidates to sign onto their plan, which is available on their respective websites:

www.GrannisForCongress.com; and
www.IrvineForCongress.org.

They also urge voters in districts across the country to insist that their candidates for office either embrace this plan or develop an equally specific plan of their own that sets forth exactly when and how each candidate plans to balance the federal budget.

A summary of the budget accompanies this press release, together with documents showing the specific funding levels proposed for each agency, the and the specific tax expenditures being proposed for elimination.

-XXX-

Appendix B: Summary of the Libertarian Balanced Federal Budget for FY 2012

Top-Level Summary of the Libertarian Balanced Federal Budget for FY 2012

	2010	2011	2012
GOVERNMENT REVENUE			
OMB Revenue Estimates	$2,165,119,000,000	$2,567,181,000,000	$2,926,400,000,000
Libertarian Revenue Adjustments			
Extend 2010 tax rates			$(592,907,580,000)
Eliminate or phase out selected "tax expenditures"			$414,218,000,000
One-time sale of gold reserves			$108,000,000,000
Libertarian Revenue Estimate			$2,855,710,420,000
GOVERNMENT SPENDING			
OMB Spending Estimates	$3,720,701,000,000	$3,833,861,000,000	$3,754,852,000,000
Libertarian Spending Reductions			
Consolidating Agencies			$(186,423,000,000)
Privatizing Programs			$(26,337,000,000)
Eliminating Block Grants			$(20,262,000,000)
Ending the War on Drugs			$(16,351,900,000)
Other Program Savings*			$(497,791,700,000)
5% Across-the-Board Cuts			$(165,034,820,000)
Libertarian Spending Estimate			$2,842,651,580,000
OMB BUDGET DEFICITS	$(1,555,582,000,000)	$(1,266,680,000,000)	$(828,452,000,000)
LIBERTARIAN BUDGET SURPLUS			$13,058,840,000

* "Other Program Savings" consists primarily of program cuts in Agriculture, Defense, Health and Human Services, State, and Transportation.

SUMMARY OF PRINCIPAL SPENDING REDUCTIONS

Consolidating Agency Functions. The idea that we can balance the budget through ten or twenty years of slow, steady dieting is unrealistic; the time horizon is simply too long and our debt burden is too heavy to give us that much time. Accordingly, rather than asking government to do more with less, we want government to do less and let the private sector do more.

Toward that end, we propose to eliminate the Department of Education, the Department of Housing and Urban Development, NASA, the National Science Foundation, the Environmental Protection Agency, and the Small Business Administration. These agencies pursue worthy goals, but government action is not the only or even the best way to meet those goals.

Privatization of Certain Functions. Many useful services provided by government are substantially similar to services otherwise provided by private entities without taxpayer support. Under this proposal, Amtrak, the Postal Service, the Federal Aviation Administration, and the Transportation Safety Administration would all be privatized.

Eliminating Block Grants to State and Local Governments. One of the greatest inefficiencies in the federal budget is the use of block grants to boss state and local governments around. This means Washington is collecting money from people all over the country and then sending it back where it came from—after taking a cut and usually attaching some conditions. Washington's instructions on how to spend the money are written by people who are never as familiar with local needs as the state and local governments are. After eliminating, consolidating, or privatizing other government functions, we would dramatically reduce the extent to which surviving federal programs serve merely as check-writing overlords to state and local governments.

Ending the Federal War on Drugs. Whether one is for or against full legalization of marijuana or other drugs, there is no good policy reason for drug prohibition to be federal and we can find no authority for it in the Constitution. Ending the federal drug war will save tens of billions of dollars

each year for federal, state, and local governments, and will restore the political control over drug policy to state governments, where it belongs.

Eliminating or Reducing Other Government Programs. Even agencies with a clear constitutional mandate for important public functions have some programs that are ineffective, unaffordable, or both. Our budget therefore proposes to eliminate roughly $500 billion in annual spending as follows:

- Over $140 billion from the Defense budget, including a $53 billion reduction in discretionary spending on overseas deployments.

- Over $130 billion in food subsidies from the Agriculture budget.

- Over $104 billion in block grant programs from the Department of Health and Human Services

- Almost $60 billion in the Department of Transportation, from terminating the Federal Highway Administration and the Federal Transit Administration.

- Almost $49 billion more in the budgets of the State Department and other international assistance programs.

- Smaller program cuts in the Commerce Department, the Justice Department, and the Labor Department.

Economizing by 5% Across the Board. Getting more selective about what we ask government to do is the key to fiscal responsibility, but there's always room for old-fashioned belt-tightening. The programs that survived our budget review will still need to stretch their resources farther, just as households and small businesses are learning to do. That 5% increment— roughly $165 billion in 2012 under our budget—would not come close to balancing the budget by itself, but as the *final* step in the process it makes our government (barely) affordable.

Summary of Spending Cuts by Agency and Category

	OMB's Budget		Our Budget				How We Did It			
	OMB 2010 Estimate	OMB 2012 Estimate	Libertarian 2012 Proposal	% Change from OMB 2012	Agency Consolidation Savings	Privatization Savings	Block Grant Savings	Drug War Savings	Other Program Savings	5% Across-the-Board Savings
Agriculture	142,016	137,917	6,329	95.4%					(131,255)	(333)
Commerce	16,714	10,430	7,242	30.6%			(690)		(2,117)	(381)
Corps of Engineers	10,536	5,879	5,580	5.1%			(5)			(294)
Defense -- Military	692,031	653,424	486,564	25.5%				(1,589)	(139,663)	(25,609)
Defense -- Civilian Programs	54,317	56,457	53,634	5.0%						(2,823)
Education	106,944	85,178	0	100.0%	(85,178)					
Energy	38,278	34,792	18,338	47.3%	(15,489)					(965)
EPA	11,301	9,980	0	100.0%	(9,980)					
Executive Office of the President	715	427	406	5.0%						(21)
General Services Administration	1,782	2,170	2,062	5.0%						(109)
Health and Human Services	868,762	911,291	762,621	16.3%			(115)	(4,285)	(104,247)	(40,138)
Homeland Security	52,903	46,847	35,350	24.5%		(5,724)		(3,798)		(1,861)
Housing and Urban Development	62,518	48,153	0	100.0%	(48,153)					
Interior	12,042	12,803	8,277	35.3%			(4,080)	(10)	(4,028)	(436)
Justice	30,333	33,700	19,311	42.7%			(4,814)	(4,531)	(7,709)	(1,016)
Labor	209,265	90,790	78,927	13.1%						(4,154)
Legislative Branch	5,423	5,292	5,027	5.0%						(265)
NASA	19,123	18,953	0	100.0%	(18,953)					
National Science Foundation	7,819	7,558	0	100.0%	(7,558)					
Office of Personnel Management	71,603	75,956	72,158	5.0%						(3,798)
Other Independent Agencies	8,427	26,915	20,648	23.3%		(3,790)	(989)	(401)		(1,087)
Small Business Administration	5,978	1,112	0	100.0%	(1,112)					
Social Security (Off-budget)	683,867	738,430	701,509	5.0%						(36,922)
Social Security (On-budget)	85,108	77,304	73,439	5.0%						(3,865)
State and Other International Programs	49,625	58,288	7,729	86.7%		(16,823)	(4,589)	(1,257)	(48,895)	(407)
The Judiciary	7,159	7,351	6,983	5.0%				(3)		(368)
Transportation	90,944	82,817	1,448	98.3%				(60)	(59,878)	(76)
Treasury	502,980	685,279	646,227	5.7%			(4,980)	(418)		(34,012)
Veterans Affairs	124,565	122,369	115,853	5.3%						(6,098)
Allowances	18,750	(4,187)	(4,187)							
Undistributed Offsetting Receipts, On-Budget	(137,793)	(150,648)	(150,648)							
Undistributed Offsetting Receipts, Off-Budget	(133,334)	(138,175)	(138,175)							
Totals	3,720,701	3,754,852	2,842,652	24.3%	(186,423)	(26,337)	(20,262)	(16,352)	(497,792)	(165,035)

Tax Expenditures Eliminated

	2012	2013	2014	2015	2016-2021	Total
Tax expenditures for corporations						
Eliminate corporate tax preferences for foreign operations	$42,920	$43,900	$43,510	$44,040	$264,240	$438,610
Eliminate corporate tax subsidies for R&D in science, space, and technology	$8,470	$8,790	$8,514	$8,878	$53,268	$87,920
Eliminate corporate tax subsidies for energy R&D and energy conservation	$15,720	$11,240	$7,080	$4,710	$28,260	$67,010
Eliminate corporate tax subsidies for forestry and mining operations	$1,620	$1,680	$1,790	$1,900	$11,400	$18,390
Eliminate corporate tax subsidies for agriculture	$40	$40	$40	$40	$240	$400
Eliminate corporate tax subsidies for financial institutions and insurance companies	$2,870	$3,050	$3,250	$3,430	$20,580	$33,180
Eliminate corporate tax subsidies for housing	$8,290	$9,450	$9,880	$10,130	$60,780	$98,530
Eliminate reduced rate for first $10 million in corporate income	$3,070	$3,150	$3,420	$3,600	$21,600	$34,840
Eliminate corporate tax subsidies for transportation expenses	$70	$40	$40	$30	$180	$360
Eliminate corporate tax subsidies for development projects	$1,390	$1,380	$1,390	$1,340	$8,040	$13,540
Eliminate corporate tax subsidies for "US production activities"	$10,910	$11,570	$12,260	$12,950	$77,700	$125,390
Eliminate tax exclusion of interest on hospital bonds	$1,420	$1,420	$1,470	$1,550	$9,300	$15,160
Eliminate tax credit for orphan drug research	$350	$380	$410	$450	$2,700	$4,290
Eliminate special Blue Cross/Blue Shield tax subsidy	$660	$590	$530	$690	$4,050	$6,520
Eliminate special ESOP rules	$1,410	$1,480	$1,550	$1,620	$9,720	$15,780
Eliminate exclusion of interest on public purpose state and local bonds	$12,140	$12,170	$12,570	$13,200	$79,200	$129,280
Eliminate miscellaneous tax subsidies for higher education	$2,320	$2,430	$2,500	$2,590	$15,540	$25,380
Subtotal	$113,670	$112,760	$110,204	$111,148	$666,798	$1,114,580
Tax expenditures for individuals						
Phase out (2 years) tax expenditures relating to foreign income of U.S. citizens	$3,615	$7,590	$7,970	$8,370	$50,220	$77,765
Phase out (2 years) tax subsidies for R&D in science, space, and technology	$165	$360	$380	$400	$2,400	$3,705
Eliminate tax subsidies for energy R&D and energy conservation	$1,250	$1,270	$1,200	$1,160	$6,960	$11,840
Eliminate tax subsidies for forestry and mining operations	$660	$710	$750	$800	$4,800	$7,720
Eliminate tax subsidies for agriculture	$830	$990	$1,130	$1,300	$7,800	$12,050
Phase out (10 years) mortgage interest deduction	$11,662	$25,568	$41,700	$59,824	$673,020	$811,774
Phase out (5 years) capital gains exclusion on principal residence	$7,902	$17,456	$28,920	$44,880	$336,600	$435,758
Phase out (10 years) property tax deduction on principal residence	$2,973	$6,268	$9,810	$13,476	$151,605	$184,132
Phase out (5 years) exclusion of net imputed rental income	$8,162	$16,408	$28,998	$44,880	$252,450	$350,898
Phase out (5 years) other miscellaneous tax subsidies for housing investments	$3,154	$7,564	$13,104	$19,848	$148,860	$192,530
Eliminate tax preferences for financial institutions and insurance and annuity contracts	$24,000	$25,720	$27,500	$29,120	$174,720	$281,060
Eliminate deduction for "US production activities"	$3,510	$3,720	$3,950	$4,170	$25,020	$40,370
Eliminate exclusion of employer-paid transportation costs	$3,820	$3,970	$4,150	$4,310	$25,860	$42,110
Eliminate tax subsidies for development projects	$1,620	$1,760	$1,860	$1,920	$11,520	$18,680
Eliminate exclusion for employer-provided health insurance premiums	$191,540	$208,650	$228,040	$248,600	$1,491,600	$2,368,430
Eliminate exclusion for self-employed health insurance premiums	$6,150	$6,580	$7,120	$7,780	$46,680	$74,310
Eliminate exclusion of interest on hospital bonds	$2,690	$2,890	$3,070	$3,240	$19,440	$31,330
Eliminate special ESOP rules	$490	$520	$550	$580	$3,480	$5,620
Phase out (4 years) exclusion of interest on public purpose state and local government bonds	$5,748	$12,365	$19,658	$27,710	$166,260	$231,740

Tax Expenditures Eliminated

Phase out (4 years) deduction for state and local taxes	$14,525	$30,945	$48,990	$68,250	$409,500	$572,210
Phase out (4 years) miscellaneous tax subsidies for higher education	$6,083	$12,800	$20,010	$27,720	$166,320	$232,933
Subtotal	$300,548	$394,104	$498,860	$618,338	$4,175,115	$5,986,965
Total	$414,218	$506,864	$609,064	$729,486	$4,841,913	$7,101,545